W9-BZL-394

MANUFACTURING SOCIAL DISTRESS
PSYCHOPATHY IN EVERYDAY LIFE

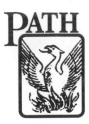

PATH IN PSYCHOLOGY
Published in Cooperation with Publications for the
Advancement of Theory and History in Psychology (PATH)

Series Editors:
David Bakan, *York University*
John Broughton, *Teachers College, Columbia University*
Robert W. Rieber, *John Jay College, CUNY, and Columbia University*
Howard Gruber, *University of Geneva*

Manufacturing Social Distress

Psychopathy in Everyday Life

Robert W. Rieber

John Jay College of Criminal Justice and Graduate Center
City University of New York
New York, New York

PLENUM PRESS • NEW YORK AND LONDON

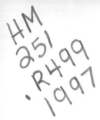

Library of Congress Cataloging-in-Publication Data

Rieber, R. W. (Robert W.)
    Manufacturing social distress : psychopathy in everyday life /
Robert W. Rieber.
        p.   cm. -- (PATH in psychology)
    Includes bibliographical references and index.
    ISBN 0-306-45346-0
    1. Social psychology.   2. Social change--Psychological aspects.
3. Social values.   4. Distress (Psychology)   5. Deviant behavior.
6. Psychopaths.   7. Anomy.   I. Title.   II. Series.
HM251.R499   1997
302--dc21   96-52872
                                                                CIP

ISBN 0-306-45346-0

© 1997 Plenum Press, New York
A Division of Plenum Publishing Corporation
233 Spring Street, New York, N. Y. 10013

http://www.plenum.com

Printed in the United States of America

This book is dedicated to my family and to all
those who have dedicated their life to the principle
"let right be done"

FOREWORD

Toward the Psychology of Malefaction

This is a book about human wickedness.

I would like to identify two obstacles in the path that this book seeks to traverse. One obstacle is an inappropriate scientism; the other is an inappropriate moralism.

There is a kind of scientism that prevents us from seeing that human beings are responsible for what happens on the planet. It is a view that, in the name of science, downplays the role of human beings as agents in what takes place.

This view is often expressed in a paradigm that regards human conduct as the "dependent variable," while anything that impinges on the human being is considered the "independent variable." The paradigm further takes the relationship between the dependent and independent variable to be the result of natural law. It characteristically ignores the possibility that individual or collective decision or policy, generated by human beings and not by natural law, is and can be regulatory of conduct.

I can best indicate the second obstacle by an anecdote. Some years ago I was invited to participate in a symposium to consider the Holocaust. I was asked to consider the Holocaust from the point of view of a psychologist. At the time, I was very interested in the history of psychology and was concerned with the radically different canon of method that the latter required. Psychologists at the time had come to the point of conceiving of the experimental method as the acme of achievement of the scientific method. History, of course, did not lend itself to study by the experimental method.

What I thought would be interesting would be to make a study of Hitler's *Mein Kampf* as a psychological document. This meant to take the writing of the document itself as a form of conduct, and attempt to make inferences back to the mind that was behind this conductor. My effort, much as that of many of the observations and speculations that Rieber cites, was to come somehow to a better understanding of the mind that was behind the wickedness we refer to as the Holocaust. Note that I have used the terms "wickedness" and "understanding" in the same sentence. My intention was that an increase in the understanding of wickedness might be a step toward preventing wickedness.

I did not fully realize that for many those two words could not go together. I certainly did not realize the extent to which my effort would offend. The very idea that anyone should try to understand Hitler in any way, understanding taken to be antithetical to condemnation, seemed to some to be an insult to the memory of those who suffered and died in the Holocaust. Hitler did not, as it were, deserve understanding. For many, understanding seemed to imply something like sympathy, apology, forgiveness, condoning, redemption, and so on. The reaction was so strong that I decided to withdraw my presentation from a printed version of the proceedings of the symposium. I was not sure that I had actually advanced our understanding that much. And I had no wish to add to the pain and suffering that had followed from Hitler's actions. I still wonder whether I did not err at that time with respect to the publication decision.

Rieber's efforts might meet these obstacles. The following observation might be made with respect to both of them.

Consider where we are in history. Our civilization began some 6,000 years ago. The great agonies of this long history, and much of the time before that, have been—perhaps oversimplifying, but not greatly—overwork and material want. Somehow, now for the first time in human history, we have come to the point where, in principle, no one need ever again suffer from overwork or material want.

The "in principle," of course, refers only to our technical capacity. For there is a vast gulf between "in principle" and "in fact."

Wickedness is one of the factors that keeps the gulf open. The closing of that gulf should be our major world project.

Wickedness is a term mostly to be found in children's books these days. Let me use another term. Let us say "malefaction," meaning the making of bad things happen, of the doing of wrong. It is a parallel term in some respects to the term that Rieber uses in the title of this book, "manufacture." Manufacture is the making of things by hand. Rieber, however, uses the term metaphorically.

Rieber's book takes malefaction as a reality to be investigated. He opens the doorway to a new systematic scientific discipline, which might rightly be called the psychology of malefaction. I cannot imagine a discipline more needed for the coming age.

DAVID BAKAN
Professor Emeritus, York University

PREFACE

This book is about the trials and tribulations of postmodern society. The postmodern lifestyle, with its current tendency to periodically reinvent itself, suffers from an unfortunate institutionalized ailment—"trained disability." Within this context, the story of the life of the mind emerges as a dialectic between in "nomine Domini" and in "nomine diaboli."

Given the free-willing nature of the life of the mind, the great book tells us that there are serpents even in the Garden of Eden. Pop culture as well as the intelligentsia seem to be telling us that today these serpents are developing an immunity to guilt and conscience, and that this immunity is spreading within world culture like a social virus. The anxiety and desperation brought about by these circumstances give rise to magical solutions, high technology, escape mechanisms, virtual reality, and (most recently) just listening to Prozac.

All around us people appear to be in dubious conflict. That is, they fear that they are being or may be victimized, while at the same time, they seek the secondary gains of victim status. In the meantime, all this is taking place in the context where social institutions that should regulate and stabilize the social order instead irresponsibly deregulate and disintegrate under the flag of freedom. An atmosphere of circus mania litigation permeates the social climate, while persons in high places attempt to assure us that they can be trusted.

In broad brush strokes, this is the essence of the subject matter of this book on psychosocial distress. A slow and satisfying insight about how we institutionalize stress began to generate in my mind in 1980. This vision was clearly the outcome of many interests that had to be clarified and connected. The dominant theme of my thinking and writing for many years has been the identification of important broken connections (i.e., body-mind, nurture-nature, cognition, emotion, and activity, etc.) that may be found in the literature of psychology in particular and the social sciences in general. The unraveling of ideas that attempt to construct a critical analysis of society at large is in any case a self-searching endeavor with many influences.

When I formally began to write this book, I was not absolutely certain of its ultimate structure. Nevertheless, the work of Eric Fromm,[1] Abram Kardiner,[2] and Gregory Bateson[3] would turn out to be an important foundation of much of my work. My personal friendship and association with Abram Kardiner and Gregory Bateson provided me with a unique opportunity to obtain firsthand information from three of the most prominent scholars in the field. Many friends and colleagues have given me the benefit of their criticisms of my ideas and early drafts and, in many instances, have offered helpful suggestions. I have given every criticism that has come my way the most earnest attention; many I accepted and made the appropriate changes. In some instances, I felt that, at some points, I was misunderstood and attempted to revise my presentation to lessen the likelihood of similar misunderstandings by others.

I owe a very special kind of debt to my friends and colleagues David Bakan, Jason Brown, Noam Chomsky, Maurice Green, Howard Gruber, Robert Kelly, Tom Langner, Robert Jay Lifton, Seymour Sarason, Herbert Spiegel, William Stewart, and Jeffery Wollock. The basic argument of this book was written in collaboration with Maurice Green and first appeared in a book that I edited in 1989 dedicated to Gregory Bateson.[4] Chapters 3 and 6 are somewhat revised versions of papers written in collaboration with Robert Kelly.[5,6] It is to be hoped that in this pragmatic critique of our brave new world, a great awakening will bring us out of our current big sleep.

CONTENTS

MANUFACTURING SOCIAL DISTRESS

PSYCHOPATHY IN EVERYDAY LIFE

INTRODUCTION

The Lay of the Land and the Currents of the River

> The immaterial self labors under the defect that it can never be perceived and understood by itself let alone the world around it.
> ROBERT W. RIEBER

> Tis the times plague, when madmen lead the blind.
> WILLIAM SHAKESPEARE, *King Lear*, IV.i

This is a book about social distress, violence, and the journey through the ever so complex terrain of the dark side of society. Social distress in postmodern America, which began with the dawning of the industrial revolution, embodies some of the greatest dangers facing us today. Given the breadth of the discussion, I first briefly describe the lay of the land I am about to explore and the underlying currents giving it life and breath.

Social distress flourishes at the very highest levels of American society as a severe and possibly self-destructive societal reaction. Its most important symptom, the psychopathy of everyday life, is a central feature in our current lifestyles. The social conditions that foster it are an indispensable part of American pluralism.

SOCIAL DISTRESS

In the language of the social sciences, the term "social stress" traditionally describes the objective disturbances in a society's

1

mode of functioning. More specifically, "social distress" refers to the inner value conflicts that arise as a society undergoes rapid changes in its basic social structure. Perhaps the most spectacular example of social distress known to modern anthropology is the case of the Ik, a tribe that was forcibly relocated to a terrain alien to its people. In only one generation, Ik economy, local organization, and customs deteriorated to the point where psychopathic behavior became the norm. The Ik may be contrasted to the Tanala of Madagascar, a tribe organized along a strongly patriarchal model in which competition was suppressed in favor of strong dependency patterns. When the Tanala were forced to adapt to a competitive economy, both homosexuality and witchcraft increased tenfold as the traditional values yielded maladaptive outcomes in the new social circumstances. Unlike the Ik, the Tanala continued to feel inner conflict about these developments. I shall discuss these two paradigmatic cases in the following chapters as I go more deeply into the causes and effects of social distress.

In today's mass society one can feel an intense increase of social distress. As the bonds of ethnicity and community have begun to weaken, the value systems of the hyphenated American have come to be detached from daily social practice. Yet in a country long accustomed to affluence, it is expected that these values will continue to be actuated by the social institutions that have always promoted them. On the contrary, existing institutions, instead of continuing to advocate and support the traditional ethical standards, are more likely to become saddled with contradictory values, to the point that they no longer function effectively. The "seven institutionalized stressors," that is, existing institutions ranging from the family to the governmental system, have become dysfunctional by being overburdened with conflicting value schemes. The modern city college, for instance, in addition to the traditional goal of imparting knowledge, has also been asked to achieve an entirely different purpose, that of offering equal opportunity to all prospective students. This has resulted in policy and procedure that have failed to accomplish their purposes.

Not only is this process self-defeating; it also adds significantly to daily stress. Consider how it might feel if during the same week one faced an appearance in court and a trip to the hospital. Both institutions, the health care system and the legal system, are designed principally to provide relief. Each system, however, has become overburdened with conflicting values. We expect our hospitals to provide both free enterprise for our health professionals and care to all who seek it. Similarly, the criminal justice system has been charged not only with administering justice but also with instituting procedural safeguards designed to protect the rights of out-groups; as a result the system has deteriorated into a clearinghouse in which rights are bargained against punishment and trial is avoided.

Particularly vulnerable to the widespread value confusion is the American family. Where formerly the family had an obvious functional value in terms of economics and the protection of the young, and could be maintained despite internal strains, in today's society the family has become secondary to the marital relationship, which, in turn, is expected to provide emotional fulfillment for the partners to an unprecedented degree. The consequences are to be seen not merely in the spectacular rise of divorce rates, but on virtually every index of social functioning, showing that the American family no longer functions as well as it did three decades ago.[1]

Such dysfunctional patterns feed one another. Values that are no longer properly achieved by a given institution are reassigned to another one, making it less functional in turn. Insofar as the family, for example, no longer properly fulfills its societal role, its traditional duties will be assigned to other institutions, such as the schools, which for their part will be expected to serve primarily as child-care providers. However, as is all too evident in the nation's urban schools, the traditional goal of providing a quality education has been sacrificed as the students and teachers face an enormous number of extracurricular problems, including drugs, guns, and AIDS. Children who were once learning how to read and write and do arithmetic are now learning how to stay away from dealers, how to avoid being shot by a fellow student, and how to put on a condom.

THE PSYCHOPATHY OF EVERYDAY LIFE

My model of social distress, that I will describe in greater detail in Chapter 1, hinges on the organization and objective and subjective cultures of the five basic levels of society, from the international level to the level of the state or nation, to that of the community, to that of the family, and finally to that of the individual. Social distress affects all levels indiscriminately, and members of all levels have developed coping mechanisms with which to integrate themselves into any given societal group. Examined from this point of view, the operation of society can be perceived as not unlike that of an organism. All members of a group—whether it be a family, street gang, corporation, government, or international organization—learn to adapt themselves to the rules that their predecessors have laid out. At times, such "obedience" is forcibly turned into a creative "disobedience." When an individual or a group, as a reaction to societal pressure brought about by social distress, learns to cope with a situation in an antisocial manner (i.e., in a way that will eventually hurt and perhaps permanently damage or even destroy the individual or the group), this individual or group is participating in a social process that results in the psychopathy of everyday life.

Such psychopathic-like behavior and its relation to a variety of possible forms of social integration will be considered later in the discussion when I come to analyze the case of the Nazi doctors during the Second World War. The antisocial behavior of chimpanzees will also be described in a context that will clarify both the significance and the limitations of animal models. Psychopaths are not always more "bestial" than average individuals. Rather, they can employ distinctively human potentials for destructively different ends. One way of understanding psychopaths is to say that they, as individuals, have usurped a position of authority and influence over the group as though they could embody the whole group itself in their person—for example, Charles Manson's classic remark when asked why he had to break the law: "I don't break the law, I make the law."

The term "psychopathy" invokes the dark side of human nature. It denotes a lack of common decency, an antisocial frame of mind beyond the reach of treatment or rehabilitation. Of all diagnostic labels available in modern psychiatry, psychopathy comes closest to the category of the demonic. Building on both historical and contemporary descriptions of the psychopath, I shall attempt in my discussion to go further than all previous commentaries in isolating the basic pathological mechanisms of dissociation, omnipotence, and pathological thrill-seeking mechanisms that play a part in the creation of such "hero" types as Oliver North as well as such infamous characters as Ted Bundy and the Hillside Strangler.

The portrait of the psychopath, which I shall deeply explore and analyze, is fundamental to my theory of social distress, since it is promoted and maintained by the social structures that concern my discussion. It is generally supposed that the psychopath is a lone wolf flourishing only in conditions of complete breakdown. We shall attempt to show the contrary—that, in fact, psychopaths typically depend on accomplices, and that psychopathic behavior has traditionally been greatly encouraged on the margins of American society. A certain degree of normalized psychopathy makes up a very basic American belief: "Never give a sucker an even break." A crucial feature of our pluralistic society fosters the coupling of group loyalty with a tolerance for the exploitation of outsiders.

Where political tolerance is coupled with intense economic competition, loyalty to one's primary reference group is accompanied by a willingness to exploit outsiders to the limit of the law. America, especially urban America, has never been a melting pot. It is more like a welding shop, or a sort of mixed salad, in which homogeneous neighborhoods juxtapose ethnic groups, a process resulting in the hyphenated American, whose loyalties are divided between the overall society and a specific reference group. The logic of intergroup competition fuels a kind of psychopathic streak within American individualism considered acceptable so long as it is directed against other reference groups and not against one's own. By becoming a "success," one vindicates not only one's own ability to excel, but also the worthiness of one's own reference group and the worthlessness of every other group. The implicit intergroup rivalry legitimizes the user of "sharp" practices in the pursuit of individual goals, no matter how destructive.

Consolidating observations from psychology, ethnology, and sociology, I shall demonstrate that the phenomenon of normalized psychopathy has intimate connections with social distress. In a society no longer sure of its basic value orientations, yet still committed to social organization on a mass scale, irreconcilable value conflicts become embedded in the day-to-day functioning of all the major institutions.

We see the results of this confusion in the daily fare of newspaper head lines, in the regular apprehension of wrongdoers in all walks of life, from television evangelists to inside traders, from defense contractors to disgraced congressmen whose behavior patterns had just the day before been not only tolerated but admired as powerful and a successful adaption to achieving the American Dream. In such a world, the consensus about behavior that might be labeled "antisocial" cannot possibly hold.

I shall then delve into the intimate connection between psychopathic trends and the American society as it is prefigured through the invocation of a social dream taken from the last century, Herman Melville's *Confidence Man*. Our own world stands repeatedly reflected in the one Melville describes: a Mississippi River showboat, the *Fidele*, steaming from St. Louis in 1856, where a variety of distinctly American characters appear, from businessmen to Indian haters, from Quakers to buffalo hunters. The prevailing rule of social commerce, announced by a sign in the ship's barbershop that reads "No Trust," elucidates the tragic reality of the American national character depicted by Melville in this world of masquerade. The confident men aboard the *Fidele* are not fictional puppets on a dream stage. Rather, they are the protagonists of an all too real allegory of the contemporary scene.

What is distinctive about our new and unapologetic confidence men—the Michael Milkens, Ivan Boeskys, Ollie Norths, and Jim Wrights—is that their criminal acts are so egregious that they can no longer be accepted as part of the normal routine. Yet these are scarcely hardened criminals in any ordinary sense, nor do they reflect criminal lifestyles in the sense of embracing "outsider" status. They consider themselves—and until they achieved notoriety, they were considered—respectable people. They have accumulated all the trappings of the good citizen's life: home, family, reputation, money. Moreover, when they are caught in flagrant illegality, they are as quick to invoke traditional American values as they are to protest that they are being unfairly singled out, because "everyone is doing it."

The prevalence of this phenomenon is astounding. A scanning of the scene in any metropolitan city in the past decade is enough to confirm it. In New York, we have witnessed one scandal after another, from Wall Street to Wedtech, from the Parking Violations Bureau to the corrupt behavior of politicians in high places. Nor is the phenomenon confined to the big city. On the national level, we have seen the regular unmasking of television evangelists, the wholesale corruption among the nation's contractors and the virtual plundering of the nation's thrift institutions.

And everywhere there is a singular lack of shame. Television preachers beg forgiveness from their flock and go on soliciting contributions. Disgraced congressmen protest that they are guilty only of accepted practice. And so forth. Corruption is scarcely a new fact of life. What is new is the bland self-righteousness of the accused and the strange apathy of the public. There is little sense of outrage about these betrayals of the public trust. Everyone seems to accept as a given that people in high places will do whatever they can get away with. Indeed, often enough, the public's real interest lies in understanding the mechanics of how these particular officials and public figures were so unlucky as to get caught, as though getting caught were the only real crime. Public posturing has become the prevailing form of social intercourse. It is hard to take a critical distance in viewing this general phenomenon, since it is everywhere around us.[2]

The evolution from marginality to normalized psychopathy will be traced in Chapters 1 and 2, which will also elaborate on the central riddle of the psychopathic syndrome. I shall develop a definition of the psychopathic personality, which results from an individual's lack of inner conflict about the violation of social norms and bonds, mechanisms of dissociation, an antisocial pursuit of power, and pathological thrill-seeking. In addition, I shall also examine the immediate social environment that contributes to and sustains the tendency toward individual psychopathy.

The aim here is to advance a critical understanding of the characteristics of social distress by taking the analysis along new pathways that explore the relationship of psychopathy to larger societal pressures, which by overburdening existing institutions with contradictory goals and expectations, have rendered them dysfunctional. The theme of social distress, developed through concrete examples of inherent value conflicts in the roles we assign our schools, court system, hospitals, and other essential institutions, underscores the emergence on a grand scale of psychopathy in our everyday life.

At each step in the evolution of the diagnosis of "psychopathy"— from the nineteenth-century diagnosis of "moral insanity" to the present diagnosis of "antisocial personality"—important descriptive features have been added, all of which contribute greatly to the contemporary diagnostic criteria for the syndrome, and which I shall review and show to be a compendium of the problem united by a few recurring features. These include the psychopath's failure to learn from experience, the enduring disregard of social responsibility, and the inability to profit from treatment. I shall then take up such established interpretive rubrics as "pathological glibness," "semantic dementia," and "the mask of sanity," and discuss them in terms of the analysis of the psychopathic personality.

Contemplating, with special emphasis, portraits of the psychopath taken from literature, such as Shakespeare's *Richard III* and Shaw's *Don Juan in Hell*, I shall examine the close relationship of psychopathy to the demonic. Considering the fact that the psychopath is commonly understood to be an intrinsically evil individual, in contrast to the psychiatric understanding of mental illness, it might be asked why psychopaths fail to have the common decency to go crazy. This problem constitutes the central riddle of the psychopathic syndrome. The psychopath's apparent inability to establish meaningful social bonds, an inability accompanied by an utter lack of distress about the situation, is certainly an enduring question for psychologists and social scientists.

The preceding descriptive presentation of the diagnosis of "psychopath" establishes the basis for a syndrome analysis stressing three major features, or "symptoms": dissociation, the antisocial pursuit of power, and pathological thrill-seeking. Each of these three mechanisms will be analyzed in terms of its operation both in normal mental life and in various forms of psychopathology. What distinguishes the psychopath from those suffering from other psychological syndromes is the unique combination of all three mechanisms. In essence, the psychopath adopts an inner psychological posture in which the "me" and the "not me" are not distinguished. Accordingly, psychopaths can shift from one identity to another without experiencing inner conflicts. Their grandiosity knows no limits and there is nothing they might not do for thrills. By the same token, the psychopath's experience of others is correspondingly impoverished. Anyone that is not "me" is devalued, considered only as a means to various ends.

The distinctive triad of psychopathic traits will lead us to an examination of the continuum of antisocial behavior. The reader will be introduced to a gallery of psychopathic characters ranging from confidence men to serial killers. Among other examples, the trial of

Kenneth Bianchi, the Hillside Strangler, will be discussed in terms of what it reveals about psychopathic dissociation.[3]

The intriguing individuals described as "adapted psychopaths" manage to escape detection by both the criminal justice system and mental health professionals. In essence, they function by making a normal lifestyle into a private "game" where they make up the rules as they go along. This attitude usually originates in the familial environment, and each of its key features are reinforced specifically by various aspects of social life. For the syndrome to become consolidated later in childhood, a facilitating social environment is required. Different patterns of pathological peer group formation, from gangs of juvenile delinquents to religious cults , also must be considered when examining the etiology of the psychopathic syndrome.

ENMITY AND THE INTERNATIONAL COMMUNITY

Having explained and analyzed my model of social distress and the psychopathy of everyday life, I shall in the ensuing chapters move on to examine certain case studies, namely, particular institutions where social distress is at work. A rather large yet barely distinguished institution suffering from dysfunctional operation is the international community and its pursuit of universal peace. In an era where the nuclear arsenal[4] poses an inexorable threat to the future of the globe, the citizens of the world invariably feel subjected to an intense level of stress that inevitably leads them to anxiety and a sensation of impending doom. When the feeling of being threatened arises, no easier target exists for channeling one's well-developed emotional energies than a well developed image of the enemy. The first half of Chapter 3 will reinterpret the psychology of war and peace by means of an explanatory definition of *enmification* as well as a survey of American involvement in wars throughout the twentieth century.

War both requires and engenders enmity between two parties, and "enmification"—the process of defining an image of the enemy—constitutes the most important psychological prerequisite for modern warfare. Charles De Gaulle made the important point that a nation cannot possibly have friends or enemies. Rather, a nation may only have a given set of interests; its adversaries and competitors being those who oppose its interests, its allies those who promote such interests. Indeed, only the citizens of a nation can have friends and enemies within or beyond their nation. Enmity can consequently only be felt on the individual level and be propagated among individuals on the societal level.

A discussion of interpretations of the psychology of enmification, including the ideas of Adler, Fromm, Trotter, Jung, and Freud, will provide the theoretical background necessary for the understanding of the conflicts examined later in the chapter. Enmification is part of a complex process involving individuals who inflate their self-esteem by concerning themselves only with their own virtues, an attitude that leads to emotional contagion of other members of the society, a virulent chain of effects motivated by the internal organization of the society itself.

Mahatma Gandhi and Martin Luther King avoided the process of enemy-making by pushing for an underlying agreement on values. As an antithesis to Gandhi's and King's approach, the process of enmification construes the opponent as implacable and menacing, a threat to survival, and incapable of sharing one's fundamental value system. Enmification reduces the "other" to a "thing" that is potentially dangerous, by thoroughly dehumanizing it. This mode of thinking is disseminated by the authorities by means of the most common information channels. Enmification fosters self-deception under the guise of promoting action. It spreads as a virus, through contact, misleading itself and its victims, and creating an image of the "other" as that of a terribly dangerous enemy against which the society must intervene because of its professed higher ideals.

Honor and the National Scene

Mark Antony in Shakespeare's *Julius Caesar* ironically accused Brutus and his accomplices of being "honorable men." In our times we have witnessed a wide variety of con men, describing themselves as honorable and moral, exculpating their tragic flaws by attributing them to a universal evil force. Such financial wizards as the characters involved in the Savings and Loan bailout and the scandal surrounding the Bank of Credit and Commerce International all seem to share the personality traits of the psychopathic individual and seem to be operating much like automatons within a larger institution. These individuals still consider themselves honorable. They, and all the other self-proclaimed victims of such institutions, are honorable men, and easy prey of a much larger evil.

The American banks of the late twentieth century have evolved into something far beyond institutions designed to safely preserve assets and investments. Banks have ceased to represent the secure system that the public was lead to believe it to be. It was deregulation during the 1980s that caused many of these institutions to overextend themselves beyond all precedent; the deepest problem lies in the fact that no one person or one institution is to blame. Operating jointly as one seriously dysfunctional system, the nation's banks have reached a point of no return, having digressed too far from their traditional role.

In parallel evolution, the news media have also become a problematic institution. Having replaced the hearth as the place for family gatherings, the news has become a product, and as a producer, it is forced to make its product as attractive as possible. Thus have society's reporters—the journalists and anchorpersons—become functionally autonomous from the society they should be reporting on. And because of the international nature of news reporting as a result of technological breakthroughs during the past 20 or 30 years, the news media have turned into the global disseminator of a new form of mass-produced culture, an embryonic yet quickly growing "world culture" with serious influence on the future world order.

Yet this world culture, novel though it may be, is already evidenced in the popular entertainment of our times. These cultural media (i.e., literature, films, cartoons, comics, and so on) provide an image of what is happening in our society and what could be done to solve it. Such social dreams reflect the degree of social distress to which the society has come. In an attempt to understand the warnings coming from these social dreams, I shall analyze the symbolic language they use. Taking my departure from Melville's *Confidence Man* and moving through television's *Star Trek* to the James Bond films, I shall explore the extent to which our contemporary social dreamers understand the underlying problems of our society, and what can be done to solve them.

The James Bond film saga is related to another important theme that I will discuss—the relationship and the interaction between organized crime and terrorism. While I do not wish to discredit the validity of the distinction between organized crime and terrorism, the realities are that organized crime groups and terrorist organizations are often intertwined, adopting each other's tactics, personnel, and operational styles. Thus to say that terrorists function from moral high ground, however appalling their practices, and that mafias pursue an agenda of personal greed and self-aggrandizement is to ignore the empirical evidence suggesting that interactive effects and suffusions of tactics, methods, and personnel—the intermingling of organizations, in short—profoundly affect their goals and identities. Furthermore, it is my contention that the acceleration of terrorism as organized crime is indicative of continuing institutionalized stress, paralysis, and fragmentation.

The rise of the psychopath as a role model—an effect of the rise in social distress in our society—will become the unifying theme of the discussion. Just as "bad" has become a word indicating positive values of strength and excitement in inner-city culture, so has the image of the cool, morally flexible adventurer become a dominant hero image for the emerging world culture. This hero motif, in turn, reflects a disturbing new social reality. In a world in which social institutions cannot function effectively, the best way to succeed is to dissociate oneself from value conflicts. The mechanisms by which this numbing is accomplished combine with prevailing social conditions to produce psychopathic behavior on a large scale. This phenomenon feeds on itself, driving out "good" as a bad moral currency, and welcoming the dark side of human nature.

1

Social Breakdown and the Social Distress Syndrome

> When in doubt tell the truth.
> Never give a sucker an even break.
>
> If the scientists have the future in
> their bones, then the traditional
> culture responds by wishing the
> future did not exist.
> (C. P. Snow, *The Two Cultures and the Scientific Revolution*)

Jacob Bronowski once remarked about Joseph Priestley that if you ask an impertinent question you may open the doors to a pertinent answer. To search for the impertinent question is itself impertinent; it is a tricky, even hard, road to follow. But this is the road we intend to follow as we inquire into the processes of how we institutionalize stress within our culture.

In trying to observe the social relations that obtain with regard to the normalized psychopathy of powerful positions, we can begin with Sullivan's observation that a promising avenue toward further elucidation of the psychopathic syndrome might lie in the study of the social relations of the anthropoid apes. Sullivan[1] proposed that the anthropoid apes show the same kind of organismic, and therefore blatantly instrumental, orientation toward social relations that is otherwise characteristic of the true psychopath. Sullivan's proposal is valuable twice over in our estimation. First, it captures something of the essence of psychopathic behavior: namely, its atavistic, nearly animalistic trust. Our own view is that the same atavistic tendency is personified in the figure of the demonic that the psychopath so closely mirrors. Then, too, Sullivan's suggestion is

13

valuable in pointing out how the psychopath fails to achieve truly human status.

This is more elusive than it might seem at first sight, for anthropoid apes have quite complex social relationships. Chimpanzees, for example, have been shown to exhibit patterns of friendship, mutual cooperation, and familial association that are quite surprisingly human. But they have also been shown to manifest horrendously antisocial behavior, including the persecution of rivals, the elimination of the sick and elderly, and, in one recent study, systematic murder. This, too, after a fashion, is surprisingly human. Where the apes differ from ordinary humans, in our view, and where they resemble psychopaths, is in their failure to experience emotional conflict with regard to these swings in behavior. Theirs is not a consistent affectivity: the murder of a vanquished rival today can follow fast upon some shared activity with that same chimp the day before. As a result, chimpanzee society is an inconstant affective affair. Judging them anthropocentrically, we see psychopathic behavior side by side with behavior that seems more sociable.

A caveat may be in order here, in anticipation of an important point that we will come to in a moment. The natural habitat of the chimps is under pressure from all sides. It may be that some of the extremes of their antisocial behavior, such as systematic murder, may embody responses to environmental stresses in interaction with an accompanying breakdown in social organization. Since it was first discovered that the suicidal swarming behavior of lemmings originated in a pathogenically altered endocrine system, itself a result of stress brought on by overcrowding and diminished resources, ethologists have been preoccupied with the role of stress in fomenting the breakdown of both physical health and social behavior in animals. Perhaps the most interesting contribution in this field is the experimental work of Calhoun.[2] Through a number of environmental manipulations, Calhoun created a variety of stressfully overcrowded situations for laboratory rats. The behavioral "sinks" had horrendous effects on the rats' physiology and on their social behavior, extending over several generations. Both dominance behavior and sexual behavior, the principal forms of "instinctive" social life among rats, became rapidly disrupted in the adults.

In one of Calhoun's experiments, a struggle for control erupted over a thickly populated central enclave in which the dominant rats quickly took over and also became the most active sexually. But they were unable to discriminate between estrous and nonestrous females, not only mating with inbussive females, but attacking and "raping" those who were not ready. Another criminal group did not participate directly in the struggle for dominance, but moved in homosexual and cannibalistic gangs and often committed homosexual rape. The life of the females was disrupted most, even though they had access to protected side cages. Half died of disturbances of pregnancy or from repeated sexual assault. Infant mortality reached as high as 90 percent: infants were abandoned and eaten. Calhoun further noted among the young who survived what he termed schizoid behavior. These rats were frightened and withdrawn, incapable of competing in the behavioral sink and wearing all the hallmarks of great stress. In the third generation, however, Calhoun observed something more startling still. Young rats who had never seen normal adult behavior grew up sleek and fat and utterly asocial in every respect; they were simply eating machines and seemed to experience no stress at all.

The role of stress in disrupting social behavior of lower animals is potentially relevant to the study of psychopathic behavior in humans. For, of all creatures, humans are both the most adaptable and the most vulnerable to disruptions in both their environment and their development. Both traits, adaptability and vulnerability, are due to the absence of built-in regulators ("instincts"). Not being born like Athena, fullgrown from the head of Zeus, human infants are shaped by their culture, their parents, and their own genetic endowments in their acquisition of coping devices and emotional responses. Many mishaps can occur during the process of maturation. Most significantly, humans are not born with a full-blown capacity for feeling. The capacity for fully socialized affective response develops only under the aegis of parental protection. Out of the child's dependent interaction with the protective parent, there arise in health the distinctively human abilities to trust, idealize, imitate, cooperate with, and have affection for another. However, there is no guarantee that this will occur.

That affectivity is not inborn but must be cultivated constitutes the greatest weakness of human society. Social controls have never been perfect, and variation in character has always been high, most particularly in aggressiveness and in the capacity for affection and cooperation. Further, in complex societies increased role specialization greatly complicates the maintenance of harmonious relationships and controls over aggression. Social complexity, moreover, can interact with variations in basic character formation in multiple ways. It is not true, however, that human flexibility is limitless and that therefore anything goes. Not only is there a greater or lesser number of human casualties in any given culture, but there are also situations in which shifting character styles interact pathogenically with historical circumstance to bring about widespread social dysfunction. One culture may adapt to stress with innovation and change; another may go under. There are vast cemeteries of dead cultures.

Among the more fortunate basic social antidotes to cultural dysfunction and to the potential abuses of social aggression are the institutions of marriage and family. Not only do they distribute sexual opportunity equitably, preventing the strong from taking all the females, but they also establish kinship structures, that basic system of social cohesion. Equally, they profit the offspring by providing stability and protection. The family also provides education with regard to accepted social patterns and in a complex society may help prepare the developing individual for an appropriate social niche. The status of the family unit is thus one of the most sensitive barometers of the success or failure of a given culture's response to changing circumstances. It constitutes, as it were, an important feedback loop with regard to social change. And when, under the impact of great stress, it becomes disrupted in its own functioning, this disruption will tend to accelerate the social dysfunction that initiated the cycle. Occasionally, the result will be a frank and dramatic increase in true psychopathology.

An excellent illustration of such a disaster is provided by Colin Turnbull's study[3] of the Ik of Uganda. This tribe was originally a prosperous, religious, kindly group of hunters and gatherers who were forced from their traditional sources of food and livelihood into the mountains. Under the impact of this enforced dislocation, all social institutions deteriorated, including the family, and in only one generation the Ik were transformed into a cold people, isolated from one another socially and ruthlessly exploitative whenever the occasion presented itself. They had become, for all intents and purposes, a tribe of psychopaths. Turnbull commented, "The lack of any sense of moral responsibility toward each other, the lack of any sense of teaming up, needing or wanting each other, showed up daily" (p. 137). (The distinguished naturalist Lewis Thomas commented on Turnbull's study that the Ik acted like separate nations rather than as members of a shared society.)

Turnbull's study certainly needs to be taken into consideration with regard to any discussion of normalized psychopathy in contemporary America. Clearly, at the extreme level the Ik appear to have reached universally normalized psychopathy. And clearly the phenomenon of increased normalized psychopathy in our society would seem to be accompanied by a general overall increase in social fragmentation. But we have to ask ourselves why it is that humans who occupy high positions, who sit at the pinnacle of intact organizations, would also be prone to psychopathic developments. It is clear that the phenomena are more complex still. Moreover, we need to keep in mind that the impact of any given set of stressors is mediated by the value patterns of society. Not all societies respond the way the Ik did. For example, Louis Jolyon West[4] found a parallel case in which people behaved quite differently. The Tarahumara tribe of Mexico were likewise forced out of fertile land into the mountains, without, however, losing their humanity in the process. West discovered them still speaking their native language and maintaining a rich cultural heritage notable for its profound affectionate bonds, its deep sense of dignity of the individual, and an aversion to violence. The social institutions of the Tarahumara, in short, were flexible enough to accommodate themselves to an equivalent stressor without the development of normalized psychopathy. Accordingly, we must ask ourselves wherein lie the peculiar vulnerabilities of the contemporary American social institutions that have fostered the startling phenomenon of normalized psychopathy in high places.

To answer this, a more pertinent example is the study by Kardiner[5] of the Tanala of Madagascar, a tribe that experienced severe stress as a result of the failure of the traditional system of rice cultivation. Under the traditional method of dry cultivation, the Tanala had simply moved to a new area every seven or eight years once resources were exhausted. By the 1920s, however, they could no longer use this method without warfare, which was ruled out by the central government. Thus the old communal tribal organization had to be broken up, and there ensued a desperate scramble for the valleys, where the wet method of agriculture could be used. The old economy had been communally governed by a college of elders and maintained by an army of docile younger sons, the oldest being exempt from labor. In the new economy, by contrast, unbridled competition and aggression were necessary and readily rewarded.

But the majority of the population of younger sons was made up of meek, obedient creatures who had been trained simply to work in the fields and ingratiate themselves with their fathers. In a crisis they had little to draw upon. The story of a typical family constellation reflects the docility prevalent in the traditional culture. Two younger sons steal two wives from their father and run away with them. The father, learning of this, sets out to pursue them, catches up with them, reclaims his wives, forgives his sons, and all return to live happily ever after. Compare this with the Greek drama of Oedipus and note the absence of guilt, murder, or retribution in the Tanala myth. The young sons needed their father's protection, and he their labor; neither could afford violence or murder, besides which, the younger sons did not possess sufficient aggressiveness to kill the father outright.

What happens to such people when they become caught up in a life-and-death struggle with starvation that requires them to adopt a competitive economic system? Unable to mobilize aggression against one another directly, they resort to that classic manifestation of repressed aggression, superstition. Everyone used magic against everyone else, and everyone feared, logically enough, that they were themselves victimized by the magic of others. A psychopathic universe, reminiscent of the Ik, came into being, but only in the imagination. To be sure, this imaginative hostility protected members of the community from mutual extermination through overt aggression. It did not, however, protect the totally defenseless and totally dependent. Infanticide became common. Another phenomenon, less easy to explain, became apparent: a spectacular increase in male homosexuality. The incidence rose to five times what it had been before the crisis; the Tanala themselves were at a loss to explain it. Here we would observe that in many animal species, including the anthropoid apes, sexual displays frequently constitute the response of weaker individuals to situations of threat as a means of indicating submission. But to this we have to add the particular

Tanalese cultural pattern: Both before and after the crisis, homosexuals were invariably recruited from among the younger sons. In short, the culturally valued pattern of submissiveness found new expression as a means of insulating a portion of the male population from the increase of threatening situations.

The relevance of the Tanalese example lies in the relatively clear way in which cultural values continued to modulate responses to a radically altered economic reality. In particular, the taboo against overt aggression and the value placed upon submissiveness continued to exert a force in Tanalese social life, even though they were currently expressed in pathological social institutions such as magic and the adoption of abnormal sexual behavior. Put another way, the same values that had long been the basis for social cohesiveness among the Tanala had in changed circumstances become the basis for practices that were observed with suspicion and chagrin. This is what Kardiner proposed to call the social distress syndrome.[6]

It is important to be clear at the onset that social distress as we are defining it is not identical with stress as that term is usually defined by social scientists. Stress, whether it affects an individual or a whole society, is typically defined in terms of objective misfortune. Social distress, by contrast, is defined in terms of value conflicts as these become embodied in social institutions. Among the Tanala, the enforced shift to new methods of agriculture was a source of stress, but the increase in homosexuality and in magical practices, things that were distressing to the Tanala themselves, constituted social distress. Once we put the matter this way it becomes clear that although social distress may follow fast upon social stressors proper, it need not do so. Social distress may as easily follow upon ostensibly benign phenomena, such as prosperity or an increase in technical knowledge or even a shift in social expectation toward greater altruism. What is determinative is not that changed circumstances be inherently stressful, but that they occasion value shifts that then become dysfunctionally reflected in the institutions that are charged with realizing them.

If we put the matter in these terms, it is clear that the United States at the present time is ripe for the appearance of the social distress syndrome, if only because there is widespread disorganization in the basic value systems of its people. To some extent, this widespread value confusion represents an exacerbation of trends that have been long-standing in American culture. In my view, Graham Wallace[7] deserves credit for being the first in this century to observe the close relation between political changes and changes in the individual's *Weltanschauung*. Veblen[8] documented the distorting influence of American economic practices on American values. Kardiner, in his *Individual and Society*,[9] took this analysis a step further, as did Fromm[10] in *The Sane Society*. Fromm's idea that there might be a "pathology of normalcy" became tied to a specific critique of the "marketing" personality as a social type. It is a matter of curiosity why this strain of social criticism has died out among social scientists in recent years, when the need for it has increased. Here we would like to revive Fromm's term, but free it from a specific typology. For in our view what has become pathological about normalcy is its embrace of value confusions.

Americans seem to be confused about basic values as never before in their history. We no longer seem quite sure what we want to define as masculine and feminine. We do not seem to be sure whether we want to preserve the traditional family as we know it or scrap it altogether for some alternative lifestyle. We cannot seem to agree whether we want our democracy to evolve more along capitalist or socialist lines as the best way of maximizing material security. We no longer are certain how to balance the claims of individual autonomy and freedom of expression against institutional prerogatives and the collective external authority of public opinion. We do not seem to know whether to value more the education or the indoctrination of the mind. We do not seem to know whether to plan for war or for peace. We do not seem to be able to understand whether crime does or does not pay. We do not seem to be able to make up our minds whether God is dead or simply hiding somewhere waiting for the millennium to come. We do not seem able to decide whether we are fighting for freedom or for bondage. Even in the social sciences we are confused as to what our basic image of humans should be, as witness the current debate over sociobiology. As Ogden Nash put it, we do not seem to be able to decide whether we are "ape-like, simian, or just normal men and womenian."

As our own individual culture merges into the newly dawning world culture, with the media serving as the instrument of indoctrination, there arises what can only be described as the institutionalization of stress. Seven institutionalized stressors can be identified:

1. Private and public sector
2. Education
3. Religion
4. Family[11]
5. Health care
6. Criminal justice
7. The media

The overall uncertainty in our value orientations, institutionalized in the seven institutionalized stressors, appear to be at least partially the consequence of recent phenomena that were, in and of themselves, much heralded and ostensibly benign: affluence, technological advance, the elimination of sexual repression, and the increased concern with social injustice all play a part. In some respects, American public opinion has become more pluralist, more tolerant, and more diversified than ever before. The converse side, of course, is that we are more uncertain about what ultimate course we should be steering. But in the best "can-do" tradition of American pragmatism, we have leapt into institutionalizing all these new values without considering their impact on existing institutions. And here we should again make mention of the hyphenated American and the traditional discontinuity between the neighborhood and the larger political and economic landscape. The reason the new, more diversified value systems of the contemporary scene could be translated into institutional policies so rapidly was that so many citizens believed that they were still insulated from such changes by the neighborhood and by the family. These citizens were wrong, as it happens, for the family and the neighborhood were simultaneously undergoing their own assault. As a consequence, it was just when many Americans had begun to take their primary identification not from the neighborhood but from larger social and economic institutions that these institutions began to shift their value orientations.[12] We have been thrown into a brave new world culture and the media have become the disseminator of its values. The result, arrived at in an incredibly short period of time, has been social distress on a vast scale. We no longer seem to know what we want our institutions to do. More precisely, we have burdened our institutions with the job of realizing multiple values, values that frequently conflict with one another. One of the author's friends, to take an example close at hand, is employed by a city university system. Most city university systems were originally set up for the purpose of providing higher education at minimal cost to the city's residents. The record of city university in fulfilling this goal speaks for itself. In the past two decades, however, to this function has been added a second one: that of ameliorating the effects of racism by guaranteeing equality of opportunity in the form of open enrollment for all who seek it. While a worthwhile value in itself, equality of opportunity conflicts with an established principle of higher education that dictates that students must be ready for the level of education they seek. Too often, the sad result of the current system is, as one colleague put it, that students who cannot learn are being taught by teachers who cannot teach them in order to guarantee them an equal opportunity to get an education. And the dropout rate citywide has reached approximately 70 percent.

Equivalent conflicts can be found in most of our important social institutions. The criminal justice system was originally designed to punish the culpable. But under the impact of reforms designed to protect individual rights, the system has become a labyrinth of procedural safeguards during just that period in our social history when crime has risen dramatically.

The health care system is likewise in shambles. The society at large cannot decide between the values of universal health care and the principles of free enterprise. We want hospitals to take in all who need them; we also want them to pay for themselves. The result, predictably, is hospitals that take in virtually everybody but only take care of those able to afford private nurses, and sometimes not even them. Value conflict is an abstract idea, clearly, but these are not abstract phenomena we are talking about. They are palpably real and they dominate life as it is actually lived in today's society.

It is the phenomenon of widespread social distress in contemporary American social life that, in my view, is to a great extent responsible for the rise of normalized psychopathy in high places. Put simply, the moral bankruptcy of individuals in positions of leadership reflects a more fundamental breakdown in the values that the principle institutions in the society are expected to embody.

Often enough the connection is entirely clear-cut. The stock market, for example, is designed to serve the economy by offering a stable institutional framework for investors and entrepreneurs to find one another. But under the impact of wildly increased government spending coupled with tax decreases for the wealthy, this important institution also has become in the 1980s a forum for amassing personal fortunes through short-term speculation in a boom market. These are quite different functions: Boesky and company ran wild exploring the discrepancy. Even more clear-cut is the institutional position of Oliver North and his coconspirators. The administration requested, and the Congress approved, a rider to the various Boland amendments that made it legal for private individuals and foreign governments to do what our government wanted to do but was barred from: aiding the Nicaraguan Contras—as though foreign governments and private individuals had it in them, without any quid pro quo mind you, to underwrite the specific objectives for the Reagan administration. Hence some of the sympathy for North: What else was the man supposed to do when he had all but been invited to break the law.

Ours is a culture that has long made allowance for a degree of discontinuity between traditional values, inculcated and embodied in the mores of the local neighborhood, and the political and social activities of what is often referred to as the hyphenated American (i.e., Afro-American, Italian-American, etc.) in the larger urban landscape. The resulting tendency to wink at successful evasions of the moral code—the psychopathy of everyday life—is as American as apple pie. The experience of value conflict is painful enough for individuals as an internal affair; it is more painful still when individuals find that such conflicts have become institutionalized and confront them externally in the form of social institutions that do not work. And it becomes completely untenable when those same individuals realize that the more successful among their fellow citizens have escaped the conflict altogether, having succumbed to psychopathic institutional adjustments.

And here let us observe that we have not begun to explore the further feedback loop constituted by the loss of the family as a social insulator. The breakdown of the family is the most ominous of all the recent developments. Not only are traditional gender roles in transition, but there is widespread abandonment of parental responsibility. Adultery, abandonment, and child abuse may be immoral, we seem to be saying, but they are not *that* immoral.

For example, recently in a prominent British journal,[13] we find the following observations regarding the collapse of the family in Europe compared to the United States. It was pointed out that in many of the inner cities of the United States, the two-parent family is disappearing. Moreover, there is a general tendency toward an escalation of the divorce rate, while the single-parent family is on the increase. Another point raised in this article is that in America, "families are valued so much that most have two of them."

Furthermore, the devaluation of fatherhood was discussed. For example, a prominent Labor representative in Parliament said, "How do you get a bloke to make a go of it with his girlfriend if the wage he can get is no more than welfare?" The Swedish response to this seems to manifest itself in their tendency to nationalize the family. Clearly, this may deal with the economic side of the problem, but it certainly does not help anything else.

This raises the interesting question, soon to be answered by the next generation, of how a child shuttled between parent and parent, between school and daycare, between one cynical social bureaucracy and another, will be able to recognize psychopathic behavior for what it is, especially in a society that increasingly devalues sincerity and tenderness and idealizes "cool" detachment and self-gratification. (A noteworthy social symptom in this respect is the relative decline in the cohesiveness of the organized crime families; modeled so closely on the family as a social organization, the criminal syndicates are lately finding it hard to recruit people who understand family loyalty.)

THE PSYCHOPATHY OF EVERYDAY LIFE

The character of American social life, with its antiauthoritarian and counterdependent emphasis, has traditionally fostered a certain amiable tendency to wink at evasions of community codes. In a bygone age, this was expressed in the general cultural fascination with the figure of the Western outlaw. Outlaws, those who lived outside the law, best embodied those traits of independent initiative and emotional self-reliance that the culture valued most. And with the closing of the frontier and the increasing urbanization of American life, the outlaw was replaced in the popular imagination by that other antisocial culture hero depicted in countless movies, the gangster.

The peculiarly American attitude toward community norms was expressed in other phenomena as well. P. T. Barnum, for example, became a legendary national figure on the basis of a magnificent skill in conning people. Did the flow of customers through the sideshow tents get bottlenecked with people doubling back to make sure they did not miss anything? Counting on a general ignorance, Barnum simply added another attraction strategically placed on the other side of a turnstile: This Way to the Egress the sign read, and off the people went to see what exactly an egress might be.

Barnum's motto was "a sucker is born every minute." W. C. Fields's motto was "if it's worth having, it's worth cheating for." Sharp practice, whether at the poker table or in the boardroom, is as American as Mark Twain. Even Huck Finn, Twain's most memorable character, can be counted, in a manner of speaking, as a juvenile delinquent. Twain's motto: "When in doubt, tell the truth."

It is worth speculating about the social and economic origins of this streak in the American national character. Emanuel Kant observed something very interesting related to this.[14] It plainly has complex roots and is no simple offshoot of frontier mentality. For if the frontier was scouted by rugged individuals, it was settled by skilled, educated European immigrants who valued community and who excelled in the mechanics of social cooperation. And the general tendency to admire certain kinds of psychopathy has increased in this century as America has become progressively more urban.[15] Consider for example the reputation enjoyed by legendary bank robber Willie Sutton. Late in his career, as he faced his umpteenth jail term, Sutton was asked why he robbed banks. His answer constituted a classic example of semantic dementia; it is also part of the American lore. Sutton replied simply, "Because that's where the money is."

Tentatively, we would like to suggest that the origins of this attitude lie in the discontinuity between local communities and the larger society.[16] As America became urban, it evolved into a nation of neighborhoods. It has justly been remarked that America was never a melting pot; it was a salad bowl. The urban landscape was a patchwork of different neighborhoods, each with its own value system. And it was the neighborhood that was the crucible of citizenship. It was here that one became socialized into a community of shared values, here that one's primary identifications were acquired. The larger urban landscape was a place where a man could go as far as luck, talent, and drive would take him. Accordingly, Americans acquired a double attitude toward the mores of society. On the one hand, they were expected to exhibit traditional values at home and in their immediate community. On the other hand, within certain limits in their dealings, principally economic, outside their own social group they were expected to be as opportunistic as the situation would allow. The split is manifest in the ubiquitous hyphen of the hyphenated American. We are Italian-Americans, Greek-Americans, African-Americans, and so forth. Knowing what is entailed on the front end of that hyphen in one's dealings with other people, knowing and taking advantage wherever possible, has long counted as an essential element of common sense. And when in doubt, tell the truth.[17]

It is the hyphen of the hyphenated American, we suspect, that allows the American to pursue success so avidly. "Making it" has always been okay, even if one had to be deceitful, ruthless, and plain crooked to do so, because making it has always implicitly been understood to be at somebody else's expense, somebody from outside the neighborhood. By making it one vindicates the worthiness of one's own group in this scheme; one has in effect championed the values of the old neighborhood.

Stepping back from the latently anomic tendency of the drive for success, we ought to be aware that the phenomenon of the hyphenated American presents a parallel to Sutherland's "selective association." What constitutes affiliation and group loyalty on one level leads to disaffiliation and potential pseudopsychopathy on another. And indeed, the phenomenon of the hyphenated American, like the level of psychopathy he tolerates and even admires, is relatively benign. The American tolerance for disaffiliated behavior, in this vein, is the flip side of American pluralism and American tolerance generally. The implicit group rivalry that underlies the psychopathy of everyday life is still to be preferred to an explicitly ruthless rivalry. Carl Jung once observed about the Swiss that they were really not a peaceful people; they had merely institutionalized their various civil wars in the form of cantonal politics. By the same token, Americans might be said to have institutionalized their own civil wars in the competition for success. Relatively speaking, this is not such a bad solution. New York City is not exactly peaceful, but it is still not Beirut. And, we might add here that the transformation of the political economy and identity of the Soviet Union into Russia has recently evolved into a unique disintegration of the Russian lifestyle that is best characterized as normalized social psychopathy, i.e., the psychopathy of everyday life.

But of late there is a phenomenon on the American scene that in my opinion is certainly not benign. I am referring to the psychopathic-like behavior of prominent individuals in high positions, in both industry and government. We are confronted by the spectacle of an Ivan Boesky, rich beyond the dreams of the average American, but intent on criminal strategies for beating the system. Boesky was caught and he was punished, but not before he had the chance quietly to sell off his ill-gotten assets at current values. This, with the full cooperation of the prosecutors, was "insider trading" on a whole new level. Then, we are confronted by the incredible performance of an Oliver North lecturing the United States Congress about exigencies of deniability. For this, North was very nearly canonized by the public, though what he asserted was that he had the right to lie to them and to their representatives. And few seemed to mind. Corruption certainly is not new; neither is recklessness in government. What is new and noteworthy is the implicit assertion that this kind of behavior is somehow okay. It may be immoral, the attitude seems to be, but it is not that immoral. And if one is unlucky enough to get caught, allowances will be made to ensure that the penalties are not too severe.[18]

In this respect, it may be that the Watergate scandal marked a turning point in American mores. From the outset, few doubted that Nixon and his immediate circle were behind the burglary; nor did anyone doubt that its motive and its sponsorship had been covered up. (We still do not really know what the burglars were after.) But, as the Senate progressed, it also became clear that, with some pruning of the staff, the administration was going to get away with it, until it was discovered, quite accidentally, that Nixon had kept tapes of all his conversations. That and that alone was his undoing. As the ensuing crisis unfolded, there were many who asserted cynically that Nixon was being unfairly hounded for doing things that others got away with, that the liberal establishment and the media had long been out to get him and now were capitalizing on the ineptitude of his staff. The terms of the discussion had shifted: Nixon should have gotten away with it; only ineptitude prevented him. Indeed, ineptitude became a ploy for commanding sympathy among his coconspirators. To his credit, Nixon did not himself take this route; he fought to the end. But some 15 years later, Oliver North pleaded ineptitude repeatedly. "The old delete button" had failed him, he explained sheepishly to the committee at one point, as though a poor grasp of computer software was his only reprehensible trait.

This is something quite noteworthy. On a spectrum of psychopathic behavior, both Milken and North were far to the normal end, and quite distant from the clinical counterpole of the true psychopath. They had homes complete with warm wives and attractive children, they were gainfully employed, they were loyal to colleagues, and so on. And yet, in quite profound ways they were behaving psychopathically. The pursuit of power, risk-taking ("I still think it was a neat idea"), antisocial attitudes ("It's a dangerous world out there, Senator"), dissociation ("deniability"), and differential association ("cutouts") all were present in their behavior. Most importantly, they showed no grasp that they had done anything wrong, save getting caught. They truly believed they should evade punishment and a surprising number of their fellow citizens agree with them.[19] The absence of guilt is remarkable and unremarked on! Indeed, such is the climate that the suicide attempt of one of North's coconspirators, Robert McFarlane, was viewed as evidence of mental disorder and not as the altogether understandable response of a career civil servant to the drastic circumstance of having been publicly unmasked as a man who broke the law, lied to Congress, and sold guns to terrorists.

Milken and North are exemplary, not unique. From defrocked television evangelists to yuppie inside traders, from Wedtech to the New York City Parking Bureau scandal, the papers daily bring us fresh reports of misbehavior by respectable people in respectable places. And, to repeat, what is most surprising about all this is not that it happens, but the attitude taken toward it, both by the principals and by the public at large. It is not that immoral, the public seems to be saying. We have here on a mass scale an example of the phenomenon described by Latane and Darley[20] as "bystander intervention," which could more properly be termed "bystander nonintervention."

In trying to explicate this phenomenon—normalized psychopathy in high places, we might call it—care must be taken to distinguish it from several related phenomena. First of all, there is the behavior of the average citizen when confronted by large, impersonal bureaucracies. A majority of Americans feel it is okay to cheat on their income taxes and cheat at cards and when playing the game of Monopoly.[21] In both instances, moreover, they are scarcely apt to feel remorse; the only sin is getting caught. Their attitude is understandable in terms of the vast disparity between the individual and the bureaucracy. The bureaucracy interferes intimately in the life of the individual's particular needs, desires, and preferences. In such an unequal contest, anything is felt to be fair. But clearly this is quite different from the sort of normalized psychopathy we have been describing. North and Boesky had enormous power; airplanes were at their beck and call, staff members went hither and yon at their command. The indifference to the prevailing social norms shown by these high-rolling players, has an altogether different basis.

If we are clear that North and perhaps Milken are not true psychopaths,[22] and likewise clear that theirs is not the understandable situation of the underdog overmatched by a large bureaucracy, then we must look to the interaction of the group and the individual in fomenting this behavior. Which brings us to the subject of the psychopathy of the group. Since Le Bon's pioneering work on the psychology of the mob, it has long been an axiom among social scientists that a group can, to a disturbing degree, inculcate antisocial behavior. Partridge[23] drew the parallel with psychopathy explicitly:

> There is another aspect of the study of the psychopathic personality ... the problem of the psychopathy of groups.... Here there is scope for much progress, and a point at which psychopathology may yet introduce methods of some precision into the wider problems of sociology. It may be assumed that within any group there is a tendency towards or possibility of the production of motives, adjustments, and behavior, which are relatively pathological: a striking and perhaps sufficient illustration is the behavior of the national consciousness, particularly in

its motivations in war. The thesis here is that the thorough and adequate investigation of the individual consciousness in its pathological
manifestation yields us precisely the background needed for the study
of the group consciousness, that is, for the development of a scientific
sociopathology. (p. 92)

Quite independently, the theologian Reinhold Niebuhr arrived
at a similar proposition in his work *Moral Man and Immoral Society*.[24]
According to Niebuhr, the paradox of modern society is that although individuals are constrained by the laws laid down by the
groups to which they belong, the groups themselves are not similarly constrained vis-à-vis other groups. A labor union must try to
get as much as it can for itself: so, too, must the company with which
it deals. Neither side can afford to extend its own standards of
compassion to the other. Moreover, insofar as one becomes identified with the group's status vis-à-vis other groups, one is encouraged to act egoistically. A union negotiator has to be ruthless if the
occasion calls for it. So do its members on the picket line.

If we stay with Niebuhr's analysis a bit longer, however, it
quickly becomes apparent that all groups must obey some set of
overarching rules if society is not to fragment completely. These
rules may not amount to moral codes of the profundity of the Ten
Commandments, but nonetheless they offer essential restraints.
Exactly here, however, the behavior of a Milken or an Oliver North
differs from that of, say, a labor negotiator. North was doing more
than representing the interests of a group within the administration;
he was breaking the rules that govern how all such group interests
are to be reconciled in the formation of policy. If North's scheme for
an independent, self-financing covert action agency had come to
pass, we would all potentially be at its mercy. Similarly with Milken:
He was not simply putting his firm's interests first; he was doing so
in a way that if it came into general practice would result in economic chaos. Given that ours is a pluralistic society and hence one
that depends on the observance of certain overarching rules, people
who break them ought to merit special condemnation. Americans of
all people ought to show special sensitivity on this point. Yet, just
here, surprisingly, we allow all kinds of things to pass.

A more permanent parallel to the current phenomenon is that
described by Robert Jay Lifton in his analysis of the Nazi doctors
who administered to the death camps. In chilling detail, Lifton[25]

depicts the inversion of values whereby killing became equated with social healing. But doctors being people and true monsters like Mengele being hard to come by, the inversion of values at the ideological level was not in and of itself sufficient. Supplementing it at the individual level were techniques of "numbing" and "doubling" whereby the meaning of the process was progressively neutralized. For Lifton's "numbing" and "doubling" we would prefer the more general, if less colorful, "social dissociation." But the essential process is obviously the same. In what sense, however, can we compare the numbing described by Lifton with the indifference of a North and a Milken? The techniques of dissociation, both individual and social, used by the Nazi doctors were necessary precisely because the conflict in values was all too palpably real. North, by contrast, seems to have been aware of no such conflict. North acquired his attitudes well before he put them into practice. Whether in Vietnam or in boot camp or someplace else, he had learned to dissociate and rationalize long before it was found necessary to support the Nicaraguan Contras.

Mower,[26] in an important theoretical discussion regarding the difference between normals, neurotics, and psychopaths, makes the following observation. Given a bell-shaped curve with psychopaths and neurotics on either extreme and normals in the middle, Mower makes the point that the therapeutic objective should be to help the patient (neurotic) move away from the position of excessive superego severity in the direction of psychopathy, but to stop somewhere in the area of normality. This assumes that the neurotic's basic difficulty is not that his conscience or super ego is excessive but that his conscience has itself been repudiated and perhaps been suppressed. Here the neurotic, rather than being overcontrolled, falls somewhere between the criminal psychopath on the one hand and the normal person on the other. The assumption here is that such a person has an essentially normal and basically adequate conscience but it has been muted or dissociated. Mower suggests a more adequate representation of this dynamic would be a J-type curve rather than a normal curve and cites Floyd H. Alport's research that demonstrated that J-type curves are very typical of social phenomena in general. Since character is manifesting a social product, we should not be surprised to come up with this finding. Furthermore, David Bakan,[27] argues that psychoanalysis has had its greatest impact not as individual therapy, as great as that has been, but as a broad social ideology, i.e., a belief system. Some also argue in this reference[28] that as a social ideology or philosophy of life, psychoanalysis has been even more mischievous than in the therapeutic process, mainly because it has in this form affected so many more people. With this frame of reference we can now better understand the dynamic, contagious process that helps produce the psychopathy of everyday life.

TOWARD A THEORY OF SOCIAL DISTRESS

Before explicitly proposing a theory for social distress, it is perhaps important that we reiterate the difference between the concepts of stress and social distress. In so doing, let us turn our attention for a moment to social stress and its impact on the individual and the society. While the term "social distress," as we have already seen in previous examples throughout this chapter, refers to the inner value conflicts that can arise in the wake of rapid social change, the term "social stress" is used to describe the objective disturbances in a society's mode of functioning. Any social system, when it disturbs basic social needs, causes stress on individuals or groups of individuals, such as families, minorities, and socioeconomic classes. Although stress understood on one level may account for acute disruptions in one's life, such as when going through a divorce or when taking a test, everyday normative stress also plays an important role when a given societal group experiences tensions that arise from gender differences, racial disputes, class struggles, and so on.

Contemporary research on social stress that does not incorporate or identify sociological variables, such as gender, race, or class, defines stress as an umbrella term that covers too much ground. A 1988 study[29] cites an estimate by the National Institute of Mental Health stating that one-third of all Americans suffer from a serious psychological dysfunction during their lifetime. While some of these dysfunctions may be caused by acute stressful occurrences in an individual's personal life, most of them are caused by the everyday normative setup of society, the influences of which seem to have malignant psychological effects on the individuals. In order to examine the specific social influences and problems stemming from systematic social practices that have such psychological effects, one must take into account different levels of stress that are provoked by the society itself and the values it imposes on its members.

Ratner[30] explains that a certain situation becomes stressful when a social need has been violated. Unemployment, for instance, is stressful in a culture where the socially accepted norm is to work and earn money. An unemployed member of the society may therefore suffer psychologically because of the stress of existing in a culture that values work and overlooks situations where one may be unable to find work. Most of the reasons for society's high rates of psychological dysfunction are connected with practices of the macrosystem, and not to the short-lived stressors such as the immediate unavailability of work. The malevolent aspects of social systems make up the foundations for enduring normative features of institutionalized inequities in power and poverty, and the dehumanizing systems of values of the society at large become the fundamental stressors.

Considering gender role as a normative societal stressor, Carol Smith-Rosenberg[31] argues that middle-class women are stressed by the contradictory role of women in their societal group. Women are supposed to be dependent, childlike, and innocent, an image contradicted by the demand for the self-responsible independent mother, homemaker, and wife. Women who fulfill the latter role are left feeling guilty and unprepared for dealing with the idealized woman. According to Grove,[32] a higher percentage of married women are psychotic as compared to married men. This finding indicates that the role of the woman in contemporary marital social relationships is more difficult to handle, that is, more stressful than that of the man.

Socioeconomic class is another normative social variable that has been found to relate to psychological dysfunctions. Research on the relation between poverty and mental illness has indicated that lower-class individuals are more susceptible to mental disturbances. Recent research[33,34,35] points out different reasons for the assertion. Working-class children lack opportunities that might help enhance their coping skills, security, and self-confidence as members of society. A member of the lower classes is not as socially accepted by the society, a fact that causes additional stress on the individual. Poorer families are at a greater risk for passing mental illness to their offspring, as suggested by various studies.[36,37] The influence of what Ratner calls "parental psychopathology" constitutes yet another aspect of lower-class deviance. It was found that parental social status was a more powerful risk factor than the presence of schizophrenic parents.

When individuals react to institutions and social structural stressors, they do so in accordance with the limits of their personality and its threshold for withstanding different amounts of stress. As for the various styles in which individuals may approach this situation, some will become totally alienated from the society while others will be ready to revolt against it. In reference to the alienation syndrome, Seeman[38] composed a model that constitutes a method for dealing with psychological and physiobiochemical stress reactions. Seeman described the topology showing the approach toward alienation. Its five components, four of which are viewed on the cognitive level and the last on the affective level, are as follows: powerlessness, meaninglessness, normlessness, isolation, and self-estrangement.

Each of these five components mitigates stress levels. The cognitive elements feed back operationally to modify psychological stress while the affective component, self-estrangement, operates to modify physiobiochemical stress. This model, however, has been criticized because of its restrictiveness. As shown above, stress is a part of social systems and not individual events. Seeman's model fails to link alienation syndrome to the dynamics of social structure, since it merely analyzes alienation in terms of cognitive states.

All five components of Seeman's alienation syndrome must be broad enough to include both cognitive and noncognitive reactions to structural stressors. If we compare Gottschalk's four categories of hostility with Seeman's components, it becomes obvious that the alienation syndrome extends itself into the affective arena. An individual may express anger openly through isolation or covertly through others. Both outward and covert hostility correspond to self-estrangement.

The term "culture" refers to the unified consistent quality inherent in the behavior of people in a particular group, the characteristics of which are reflected or expressed in almost every sphere of activity and interpersonal relations. The social character of a group is the element that shapes the members of society to act in accordance with cultural requirements. The society shares energy, motivation, ideas, and ideals, and is structured by economic, political, and cultural realities. When external conditions change at such a rapid rate that they no longer fit the traditional social character, that is, when there is no longer consistent behavior within a particular group, there is a disintegration, a breakdown of the social character.

The nineteenth century produced a social character whose inner drive met the social necessity for punctuality and orderliness, saving, stability, and authoritarian principle. Character structure made all members of society shape their behavior according to their economic purposes. In the twentieth century, however, we have based our economy on the fullest development of consumption and have learned to govern by eliciting consent rather than obedience. The social character of our century has developed a powerful weapon, the use of which has resulted in an erosion of the traditional social character such that the elements that used to bind the society together, the ingredients of our "social mortar," have slowly and subtly evolved into ingredients for "social dynamite." It is important to understand this process in terms of degrees. The twentieth-century Americans, for example, allow the economy to shape their behavior even more than did nineteenth-century Americans.

Within the culture there exist five ecological environments that make up the basic structure of the model we propose for psychosocial distress (see Table 1.1). The first level is that of the individual, whose subjective culture consists of a negative self-image leading to "upset" feelings, and whose objective culture consists of physical signs of depression and sickness. The second level, that of the family, subjectively produces marital and family conflict and crises of faith; objective signs are familial abuse and divorce. The community makes up the third ecosystem or environment. Subjectively there are group conflicts and feelings of prejudice within the community, and the objective reality is evidenced by job loss and decaying neighborhoods. The fourth level is that of society, which subjectively feels disenfranchised and objectively suffers from high unemployment and low voter turnout. The final level is the political structure of international relations. Subjectively nations trust each other less and less, resulting objectively in international terrorism and war. The subjective and objective cultures are correlated by psychosemantic social learning processes of attitudes, beliefs, values, social

Table 1.1
Schematic Representation of Social Distress:
Subjective by Objective Cultures at Five Ecological Levels

	Subjective	Objective
Individual	Negative self-image	Sickness
	Feeling "upset"	Physical signs of depression
Family	Marital conflict	Familial abuse
	Criris of faith	Divorce
Community	Group conflicts	Job loss
	Feelings of prejudice	Decaying neighborhood
Society	Feeling disenfranchised	High unemployment
		Low voter turnout
Political	Low trust in other nations	International terrorism
		War

Note: This model was developed in collaboration with Dr. Oliver Tzeng of Purdue University for empirical research purposes.

norms, tolerance, habits, behavioral dispositions, and so on, which are acquired at all environmental levels.

The psychopath has, over a long period of transitions, become the role model for this psychosemantic process. Psychopathy stands in opposition to cognitively based adaptive behaviors. As an outgrowth of a very complex, slowly disintegrating social structure, the psychopathy of everyday life feeds on alienation and anomie, picking confused individuals as easy targets. The psychopathy of everyday life is one of the symptoms of the emergence of a crisis, either cumulative or abrupt, that is perceived as beyond the normal range of social norms, ideas, or expectations and that results in conflict. The threat of this crisis will have a negative impact; it will be perceived as something beyond the control and coping ability of the individual or the group. The coping behavior intention, in contrast to cognitive reactions such as normlessness or powerlessness, is based on attitude and affective rationalizations. Eventually, it results in socially undesirable behavior such as substance abuse or violence.

Social distress is increasing in today's mass society. As the bonds of ethnicity and community begin to weaken, the value systems of the hyphenated American have come to be detached from daily social practice. However, in a country long accustomed to affluence, it is nevertheless expected that existing institutions become saddled with additional values, many of them contradictory, to the point where they no longer effectively function. In a world in which social institutions cannot function effectively, the best way to succeed is by numbing oneself to value conflicts. The mechanisms by which this numbing or dissociation process is accomplished then combine with prevailing social conditions to produce psychopath-like behavior on a greater scale. It is the aim of the following chapters to examine the social distress, as well as the psychopathic syndrome, and how it is institutionalized, along with its malignant effects within the society at large.

2

The Prince of Darkness and the Heart of Darkness

The serial murderer's dilemma: Is it
worse to be wanted for murder than
not to be wanted at all?

"After all," as Miss Beauchamp used
to say, referring to her different
dissociated personalities, B1, B3, and
B4—the saint, the devil, and the
woman, "they are all myself." And
perhaps after all, Miss Beauchamp
was not so very much unlike the rest
of us.
Morton Prince, April 28, 1915[1]

Of all the recognized psychiatric syndromes, that of the antisocial
personality, or psychopath, presents perhaps the greatest number of
unsolved questions. Although it has long been recognized that each
of us possesses an innate capacity for momentary dissociation vis-
à-vis the accepted value systems of society, and thus in that degree is
potentially psychopathic, true psychopaths—with their consis-
tently antisocial behavior—present the average observer with a
phenomenon so spectacularly alien that it seems almost incredible
that such people can exist. And granted that psychopaths do indeed
exist, it is perplexing how they can manage to appear superficially
sane, how they are able to wear, as one observer put it, the "mask of
sanity." The true psychopath compels the psychiatric observer to
ask the perplexing, and largely unanswered, question: "Why
doesn't that person have the common decency to go crazy?"[2]

Given the mixture of awe, horror, and perplexity that the true psychopath evokes, it is perhaps not surprising that research into the etiology, course, and psychological mechanisms specific to this syndrome has lagged far behind that of other psychiatric classifications. When we have such difficultly grasping the essentials of the presenting picture, we can only have greater difficulty in finding an overall interpretive scheme around which to organize our research questions. Indeed, we know far too little about how the psychopathic character structure comes about, how it utilizes social experience to perpetuate its fundamentally antisocial outlook, and how it often manages to secure highly stable social niches in which both accomplices and subgroup prestige can be found.

Psychopathy Today

For purposes of this discussion, the term "psychopathy" is to be preferred precisely because of its wide range of meanings in ordinary parlance.[3] For what we will presently be concerned with is a whole continuum of behavior ranging from what might be called "normal psychopathy," or "pseudopsychopathy," all the way to the horrific extreme represented by the "antisocial personality," or "true psychopath." Cleckley pointed out as early as 1941, in his *Mask of Sanity*, that each of us possesses in rudimentary degree the distinctively psychopathic capacity not to respond to the salient moral or social requirements of a situation. A gang of unruly 12-year-olds cutting up during a school outing to Carnegie Hall to hear Mozart are behaving psychopathically, notes Cleckley, as are we all when we momentarily break ranks with our conscience to laugh at what we otherwise hold in highest reverence. Nor is such a capacity intrinsically bad. To paraphrase a point made by Cleckley, were it not for this ability to break ranks with our conscience occasionally, we would all be in danger of turning into pompous monsters of self-righteousness.

This said, it is important that we first acquaint ourselves with the extreme pole of the continuum occupied by the "true psychopath." This term indicates something more than a tendency to care about others only as means to one's own self-centered aims; it indicates a *lack of capacity* to do otherwise The true psychopath is lost to humanity, utterly incapable of human concern and involvement with others except at the most superficial and exploitative level.

It is important to distinguish the true psychopath from the career criminal, at least as an ideal type. (There is plainly overlap.) Career criminals rely on superior and cunning to gain wealth; they feed their ego on the fear they evoke and on their own ability to get things "done" outside the encumbrances of the law. Nonetheless, such people are quite capable of feeling empathy and concern for their immediate family and for their partners in crime. Moreover, they rely on the support of others and are capable of erecting and adhering to quite formal procedures for inclusion within the peer group. They are concerned with winning admiration and praise from their criminal partners, and they speak in derogatory and contemptuous terms of their victims. In short, they manifest salient characteristics of group identification and group loyalty. True psychopaths, by contrast, are typically a bust even as members of an organized criminal ring; they cannot be relied on, they make unnecessary trouble, and though they may be useful for carrying out specific acts of an usually unseemly nature, there is no question of obtaining their long-term loyalty. When trouble arises, the psychopaths are the first to go, something that career criminals understand and for which they typically plan expeditious means. (New York City police are still investigating the murder in a midtown Manhattan restaurant of one Irwin Schiff, wheeler-dealer and con man extraordinaire; the further the investigation proceeds into the incredible trail of extortion, bribery, and swindles that is this man's sole legacy, the harder it has become to fix a single motive for his death. Seemingly everybody who ever knew him, including career criminals and ordinary businessmen, had something to gain by killing this man.)

Some progress in portraying the psychopath at a phenomenological, descriptive level has been made in the fourth edition of the *Diagnostic and Statistical Manual of Mental Disorders* (DSM-IV) of the American Psychiatric Association.[4] Among the diagnostic criteria needed to merit a diagnosis of antisocial personality, the essential feature is a pervasive pattern of disregard for, and violation of, the rights of others that begins in childhood or early adolescence and continues into adulthood. We have here a catalog of human evil.[5] For this diagnosis to be given, the individual must be at least 18 years old (Criterion B) and must have had a history of some symptoms of conduct disorder before age 15 years (Criterion C).

The summary of the diagnostic criteria of antisocial personality disorder in the DSM-IV is as follows:

> There is a pervasive pattern of disregard for and violation of the rights of others occurring since age 15 years, as indicated by three or more of the following.
>
> 1. Failure to conform to social norms with respect to lawful behaviors as indicated by repeatedly performing acts that are grounds for arrest.
> 2. Deceitfulness, as indicated by repeated lying,[6] use of aliases, or conning others for personal profit or pleasure.
> 3. Impulsivity or failure to plan ahead.
> 4. Irritability and aggressiveness, as indicated by repeated physical fights or assaults.
> 5. Reckless disregard for safety or self or others.
> 6. Consistent irresponsibility, as indicated by repeated failure to sustain consistent work behavior or honor financial obligations.
> 7. Lack of remorse, as indicated by being indifferent to or rationalizing having hurt, mistreated, or stolen from another.

The interpersonal difficulties these people experience and the discordant modes that they suffer persist far into midlife and beyond, even though their more flagrantly antisocial behavior, most especially assaultiveness, typically begins to diminish by the time they pass 45 or 50 years of age. Invariably there is a markedly impaired capacity to sustain any kind of lasting, close, normal relationship with family, friends, or sexual partners. Such individuals, in fact, generally cannot become independent, self-supporting adults without persistent criminal activity. However, some who warrant this diagnosis are able to achieve some degree of political or economic success—the "adaptive psychopaths"; to outward appearances their day-to-day functioning is not characterized by the impulsivity, hostility, and general chaos that typify the general syndrome.

The problem of the adaptive psychopath is especially elusive, since such people come to psychiatric attention late and only after they have run seriously afoul of the law. (And an indeterminate number of them, an elite subgroup, have simply never been caught; thus, they have never been examined psychiatrically.) Accordingly, it is impossible to get a clear picture of how they functioned during their period of ostensibly normal adjustment. Apparently, whether by virtue of superior endowment or because their survival was facilitated by adopting an outwardly compliant facade, their educational development was substantially less hampered than is typically the case. Theodore Bundy,[7] the notorious serial killer who was executed in Florida in 1988, had attended law school and become active in California politics. His truly horrifying career as the nation's most prolific serial murderer was incomprehensible to many who knew him during this phase of his life, though even then his temper was considered hair-trigger. Nonetheless, it should be observed that, although the enigma of the adaptive psychopath remains largely unsolved, such people are known to show certain hallmarks of the general syndrome, most especially the characteristic search for thrill-seeking through dangerous behavior, an attitude of omnipotence typically expressed in a feeling that they will never get caught, and a dissociative capacity that among other things enables them to demarcate periods of frankly antisocial behavior from their "normal" periods.

We might note in passing how many of the points raised in previous diagnostic schemes are echoed in the contemporary diagnostic criteria. Thus the DSM-IV subdivides the prodromal phase of a childhood "conduct disorder" into four subdivisions: unsocialized aggressive, socialized aggressive, unsocialized nonaggressive, and socialized nonaggressive. The first and third of these subgroups clearly invoke two of Henderson's subgroups, his aggressive and inadequate types. Then, too, the early onset of the syndrome—before age 15—coupled with the typical, though not invariant, lack of educational achievement is suggestive of the heredity taint of older systems; this observed lack of achievement would superficially appear to be linked to a general incapacity in intellectual functioning. (The elusive adaptive psychopath, meanwhile, is reminiscent of the genius-criminal of Nordau's typology.) Moreover, such a finding has no status in the contemporary diagnosis, per se, Henderson's observation of frequent nonspecific brain abnormalities continues to be borne out with observations on a portion of this population. And finally, the overall lack of concern with others, manifest in every facet of life, coupled with the remarkable failure to learn from experience, is indeed suggestive of an intrinsic defect for which "moral imbecility" is an altogether apt term. As for the implicit realization of the Royal Commission on the Feeble Minded that *all* treatment proved ineffective, this too has been confirmed by subsequent clinicians. Harry Stack Sullivan[8] summed up his experience thus:

> I am afraid I cannot overcome my conviction that the real psychopathic personality is a very serious miscarriage of development quite early in life, so grave that it makes a very favourable outcome possible only with an almost infinite amount of effort, which in turn, I guess no one will ever be worth. By and large, I expect to find the psychopathic personality already clearly marked off, and expect it to continue without any great change except for a slow increase in the amount of hostility that it engenders in others and the bitterness and sometimes alcoholism, which it engenders in the person himself. (p. 360 n.)

THE MEPHISTO SYNDROME

In what follows, I will attempt to identify the salient characteristics of the psychopathic syndrome with a view to establishing a taxonomy of psychopathic processes. Several points need to be made at the outset. I am far from believing that the underlying cognitive, conative, and emotional processes described below are unique to the psychopath; rather I believe in the first place that they represent gross exaggerations of tendencies to be found in everyone and in the second place that even in their pathologically exaggerated form they are not unique to this syndrome. (For example, the kind and quality of dissociative processes exhibited by the psychopath can also be found in multiple personality.) No; what is unique to the psychopath in my view is the combination of these processes; it is the combination that discriminates true psychopathy from other syndromes. This said, it should also be noted that much research still needs to be done, particularly in the areas of potentially predisposing neuropsychological factors and etiologically significant environmental variables.[9] It is enough for my purposes if the following discussion captures some of what is essential to psychopathy and does so in a way that allows meaningful generalization to what I term "the psychopathy of everyday life."

Let me begin at the level of discriminating characterological traits and then subsequently work my way down to the underlying processes.[10] In my view, the following four salient characteristics—

thrill-seeking, pathological glibness, antisocial pursuit of power, and absence of guilt—distinguish the true psychopath.

Thrill-Seeking

These people habitually rush in where angels fear to tread. The more dangerous an undertaking, the more irresistible it becomes.[11] This behavior cannot be classified as merely impulsive since it often entails planning and in a surprisingly large number of cases the cooperation of an accomplice. But such planning as does occur does not mitigate the element of danger. There is some evidence to suggest that psychopaths have unusually high thresholds for perceptual stimulation. Certainly, their overt behavior suggests that only in situations of threat and danger do they feel truly alive. The world of predictable cause and effect, of instrumental acts and expectable rewards, has no emotional meaning to them; they grasp that this humdrum, predictable, and boring world exists, but cannot relate to it. (Adaptive psychopaths have taken this to a paradoxical extreme: They can go about their routine duties precisely because they have turned them into a dangerous game of charades, of passing for normal, while in their off-hours they live an entirely different life.) Much of what has been observed, by Sullivan and others, of the psychopath's inability to learn from experience has to be related to this characteristic: Life would be less dangerous, and thus altogether less fun for psychopaths, if they really allowed themselves to "learn" and thus to "know" the altogether likely consequences of their behavior. True psychopaths prefer an open-ended world: Whether they take off in their car cross-country with no planned destination or time of arrival, or merely say something shocking and outrageous in conversation, they are seeking to create situations of ambiguity and potential danger.[12]

We might pause here to distinguish psychopathic thrill-seeking from the pursuit of excitement used by normal people to offset boredom. On a continuum of thrills, one might rate tennis relatively low and ice hockey, with its sanctioned violence, relatively high. But for true psychopaths even ice hockey is boring; there are too many rules. Psychopathic thrill-seeking consists in breaking the rules, whatever they might be, or else in surreptitiously making up new rules. At a poker table, psychopaths do not want to win; they want to cheat and get away with it. That is, they want to turn the game into a new game, where they make the rules. These people invariably rush in where angels fear to tread; theirs is the "Mephisto Waltz" on the tightrope of danger.

Pathological Glibness: The Manipulation of Meaning in the Communication of Deceit

Psychopaths invariably speak well, colorfully, persuasively, and volubly about themselves and their past (though only minimally about their future). What is said, however, has no discernible relation to facts. There is a kind of "semantic dementia," as Cleckley[13] has termed it. Cleckley's point was that the ordinary emotional demands of a situation make no impression on psychopaths; like rowdy schoolboys at a concert, they behave as if the accepted meanings of a situation simply were not there. But the same dissociation is also manifest in their speech; words have become detached from meaning and serve instead as a means of placating a dangerous foe or of fleecing an unwary victim. By the same token, they do not allow themselves to be moved by words and concepts that their fellow citizens value. Consider the psychopath who was asked, out of the interviewer's exasperation, did he not have any compassion for his victims. "The only place you find compassion," the interviewer was told, "is in the dictionary between 'shit' and 'sucker.'"

It is sometimes said that pathological glibness is to be found only in intelligent psychopaths. To the contrary, what distinguishes intelligent psychopaths is their greater productivity and their greater effort at maintaining consistency. The basic trait, however, can be found at all levels of intelligence within the syndrome. Thus my experience with an institutionalized, borderline-retarded psychopath: Having just raped a fellow patient, this fellow promptly accosted me at the door of the ward with a moving tale of woe about how the attendants were planning to gang up on him for no good reason.

Antisocial Pursuit of Power

Not only are psychopaths extremely sensitive to power relationships and extremely interested in obtaining maximum power for themselves, but they seem hell-bent on using power for destructive ends.[14] Only in paranoid states and in the attitudes of career criminals can a comparable fusion of antisocial trends with the power drive be seen. It is as though, for psychopaths, power can be experienced only in the context of victimization: If they are to be strong, someone else must pay. There is no such thing, in the psychopathic universe, as the merely weak; whoever is weak is also a sucker, that is, someone who demands to be exploited. Thus, when inmates seized control of the New Mexico State Penitentiary some years ago, they engaged not only in murder but also in mutilation of selected victims. Afterward, one of the suspected ringleaders was interrogated at length: While being careful not to incriminate himself, he made it clear that the victims of the uprising "didn't understand morality." He also made it implicitly clear that he and his cronies ran the prison anyway and that, apart from the freedom to leave, they enjoyed every advantage they had enjoyed on the outside. The prisoners, given room to maneuver by legal reforms designed to safeguard their rights, had in effect created a psychopathic universe in which the strong preyed on the weak in the name of "morality." To be sure, the fusion of the power drive with antisocial trends in the psychopath need not always be so bloodthirsty (violence per se is not a distinguishing trait of the syndrome). Consider the young man who explained that he stole cars because it was the only thing he was good at—and everyone needs to be good at something.

Absence of Guilt

Psychopaths are aware that certain people at certain times will bring punitive sanctions to bear against them. Accordingly, they are skilled in evasion and rationalization. Some, gifted histrionically, can even feign remorse. But they do not feel guilt. The absence of guilt is essential to the syndrome for, as is immediately apparent upon reflection, guilt, besides a consequence of certain acts in normal people, is also a powerful deterrent against committing those same acts in the future. Psychopaths are undeterred; indeed, just those salient characteristics that to others would portend guilt as a consequence, to psychopaths portend the excitement of danger. And when psychopaths are caught, they are in a profound sense uncomprehending. Moreover, when one investigates the absence of guilt clinically, one discovers a general poverty of affective reactions. The young man who stole cars could distinguish only two feelings in himself, boredom and inadequacy; all other feelings were "for suckers."

If we combine these four characteristics—the absence of guilt, the antisocial pursuit of power, superficial glibness, and thrill-seeking—we have what might perhaps best be called the "Mephisto Syndrome." Indeed, it is hard to resist the impression that the true psychopath is a personification of the demonic. Since time immemorial, humankind has outlined in figures of the demonic an inherently human capacity to fuse despair and drive discharge in an antisocial posture; the devil has always been important to humans as a personification of what, as intrinsically social creatures, they cannot afford to be. But it is precisely the inhibiting sense of being intrinsically social—Adler's capacity for social feeling—that psychopaths lack.[15] They are not social, only superficially gregarious; not considerate, just polite; not self-respecting, only vain; not loyal, only servile and down deep they are really quite shallow. In a word, they are fundamentally asocial beings. Hence the observed homologies with the figures of the demonic: The psychopath is free to be what ordinary humans dare not be. For ordinary humans, the figure of the devil is always experienced as a projection, as something outside the ego.[16] For the psychopath, the demonic is a way of life. Moreover, just as the devil has evolved through the centuries and has in the process of that evolution acquired a whole host of representations ranging from the truly bestial all the way to the suave silk-clad sophisticate of the comedy *Damn Yankees* and the philosophical troublemaker of George Burns's portrayal in *Oh God, You Devil*, so too can the presenting facade of the psychopath range from the grotesquely animallike all the way to the sweet-talking confidence man.

Indeed, since like the devil psychopaths are inherently asocial, they are difficult to comprehend within the confines of ordinary human morality. From a theoretical point of view, the true psychopath, like Lucifer, goes beyond the categories of evil and sin; theologically, the true psychopath is incapable of forming any relationship to God or to humans. These are the souls who reside in Dante's Inferno, these the damned of Jonathan Edward's theology. Not feeling remorse, psychopaths enter the confessional, as they enter psychotherapy, only when it serves some other purpose, typically that of evading punishment.

To be sure, such visitors from another moral world are intrinsically fascinating. We can see this in our daily papers. A Bundy or a Bianchi (the "Hillside Strangler") is the stuff of tabloid headlines and made-for-television movies. But here tabloid writers, on the whole, lack the psychological depth to explore their material past a few sensational details plus the inevitable body count. A detailed portrait of the psychopathic mind requires genius, and one should consult either Shakespeare's *Richard III* or George Bernard Shaw's dramatic sequence "Don Juan in Hell." (Such are the exigencies of the material, incidentally, that both plays require great acting to come alive. Only an Olivier, or a George C. Scott, can make the audience believe that having killed a woman's father and husband, Richard now proposes to seduce her while simultaneously admitting to his crimes. Psychopaths would consider this a challenge worthy of their grandiosity; most mortals, and most actors, consider it a plain impossibility and thus an unplayable scene.)

But if we can set aside our fascination, we must ask ourselves what are the ordinary human psychological processes at work in the psychopath that generate this personification of the demonic. Let us begin with the antisocial pursuit of power, taking as our point of departure an idea of Gregory Bateson's. Bateson has proposed a distinction between symmetrical and complementary interactions.[17] In symmetrical interactions, a given behavior leads to the same behavior in the other, which in turn becomes a signal for an increased amount of the triggering behavior of the first. Situations of mutual threat are an example of symmetrical interaction. In complementary interactions, however, the behavior of one participant evokes a reciprocal behavior in the respondent; dominance, for example, evokes submission. If we ask what exactly constitutes power in this frame of reference, it is immediately clear the power resides not in the individual but in the system of complementary interactions that identify that individual as dominant within the group. The power of the dominant individual resides in the group. Power, in short, is an abstraction pertaining to complex group processes: "It is not so much 'power' that corrupts as the myths of 'power.' ... 'Power' like 'energy,' 'tension,' and the rest of the quasi-physical metaphors, are to be distrusted and among them 'power' is one of the most dangerous. He who covets a mythical abstraction must always be insatiable!"[18] To be distinguished from the power of any individual within the group is the power of the group itself, whether it be family, community, political faction, social-economic unit, or nation. The power of the group is real; if properly organized the group can accomplish things well beyond the power of any individual. The individuals, for their part, participate in the exercise of group power through identification. And this identification is likely to be all the stronger when the group is behaving aggressively toward another group. Every fall, stadiums around the country fill up with people rooting passionately for their favorite football team, a blatant, altogether normal occasion in which an identification with a powerful and aggressive group, be it the Oakland Raiders or the Duke Blue Devils, can be safely indulged.

Psychopaths, by contrast, appear to situate themselves altogether differently vis-à-vis the group. Rather than adopt a posture of identification, they appear to act as though they believed that their relation to the group were emulative and complementary. That is, they seem to proceed on the delusory belief that in their own person they can emulate and create the degree of power that, properly speaking, only the group has. More than a law unto themselves, psychopaths act as if they were a whole nation unto themselves. Charles de Gaulle once observed that a nation has no friends, only interests. So it is with psychopaths. And their participation in the interior network of complementary and symmetrical relationships within the group—the only true dominance for the individual—is correspondingly falsified by this underlying delusion. The psychopath has collapsed the two logically distinct levels of meaning. (In passing I note that I plan to investigate psychopathic individuals with the semantic differential scale developed by Charles Osgood;[19] the prediction is that in their affective judgments psychopaths will tend to collapse the first two dimensions of the scale, evaluation [good/bad] and potency [strong/weak], into a single overall dimension. An appropriate term for this collapsed psychopathic dimension, if it proves to be detectable, might be the inner-city slang epithet "bad," which means strong, exciting, and therefore admirable; in inner-city usage, "bad" can be applied to both friends and enemies without change of meaning.)

One can only speculate on how the psychopath's profoundly disordered orientation to issues of power and social intercourse comes about diachronically. It must be somehow characteristic of the pathogenic milieu that levels of meaning pertaining to the group—its cohesiveness, stability, and continued survival—have become contaminated with levels of meaning pertaining to relations between individuals. When Bianchi, the Hillside Strangler, was seen in a child-guidance clinic at the age of 11 for school problems coupled with somatic complaints, the psychologist who examined him, Robert Dowling, noted: "It would appear from Kenneth's viewpoint that his mother has related to him in such a way that he feels his very survival depends on his being in her good graces."[20]

Here we should perhaps touch on a concept derived from the study of juvenile delinquency, Sutherland's concept of "differential association." Working out of the Chicago School of Sociology, Sutherland sought out the social causes of juvenile delinquency. Sutherland proposed that membership in an antisocial group, the gang, was necessary to incubate antisocial behavior. Clearly, the overall social structures must also tolerate this pattern or at least not interfere with it. Thus, Sutherland's thesis was supplemented by Merton's[21] concept of social breakdown, or anomie, as a contributory variable. By associating differentially with a gang, in other words, delinquent adolescents insulate themselves from the larger social network and from its rules. Differential association, in short, entails social dissociation. The group perception protects the individual from experiencing conflict.[22] Just how deeply a socially patterned delusionary system can go can be seen in the Pentecostal sect described in the book *When Prophecy Fails*.[23] The sect in question had gathered in the desert for the end of the world; when this did not occur, the leader rechecked his calculations and told the group that a mistake had been made and the end was still 50 years off. The group went home satisfied. Thus, the self-fulfilling prophecy was readjusted and homeostasis was reestablished.

Sutherland's delinquents were not necessarily psychopaths, but it is plain that some similar mixture of associative and dissociative processes is relevant to the psychopath. What delinquents do by way of distancing themselves from the norms of the community, psychopaths do at a far deeper level. And here we come to the topic of dissociation as a clinical phenomenon. Dissociation is a critical cognitive process in psychotherapy. It is manifest in the pathological glibness, in the inability to feel guilt, in the inability to profit from experience, and in the semantic dementia, generally, of the psychopath.

We ordinarily conceive of dissociation as a hysterical trait.[24] In this context, dissociation refers to the tendency of individuals to separate, or dissociate, their "real" selves from their "public" selves. Such people histrionically alter their public presentations to create a succession of socially acceptable images or facades. Dissociation thus serves as a mechanism for distracting others from the unpleasant realities that may constitute the real self. And it can reach the point, spectacularly manifest in multiple personality, where it constitutes a self-distracting process so powerful that it utterly prevents the individual from experiencing and integrating painful thoughts or emotions. At a less severe level of disturbance, the charming, dramatic, or even seductive facade of histrionic personalities prevents them from dwelling on the inadequacies that they may possess, inadequacies that nonetheless are available to consciousness if histrionic personalities are sufficiently motivated to deal with them.

With psychopaths, dissociation reaches to a deeper level; paradoxically, it is also more readily put at the service of the pathologically inflated ego. Where the histrionic splits off the "bad me" from the "good me," to use Sullivan's terminology, the psychopath's internal split seems to take place at an even more basic level, that of the "me" and the "not me." In a double sense, in both fantasy and reality, there is nothing that is "not me" for psychopaths. There is no limit to the grandiosity of their fantasies; likewise there is no limit to what they might do. And given that "me" and "not me" form a continuum of meaning, with each necessary as a semantic counterpole to the other, the inability of psychopaths to arrive at a "not me" self-structure results in a corresponding inability to arrive at a stable sense of "me" as well. (To avoid misunderstanding, let me make clear that though I speak of a stable self-structure, I do not conceive of the self as an entity, but rather as a system of interlocking processes that link the individual to the social milieu.)

Paradoxically, the deficit in self-structure or concept of the psychopath at this most elemental level is coupled with a greater capacity for the techniques of dissociation at the higher level of "good me" and "bad me." Whereas for the multiple personality, and for the hysteric generally, dissociation is primarily an unconscious process. The beauty of it is that it primarily works outside of awareness for the psychopath. There is a definite ego-involvement in it, at least insofar as social judgments are concerned. Psychopaths are constantly on the lookout for ways of distracting the interviewer, of rationalizing their behavior, of deflecting the blame. They show both foresight and perspicaciousness in forestalling any confrontation with the "bad me." They know what they are doing.

We must be careful not to confuse levels here. Because at the level of the "bad me" psychopaths manifest a degree of conscious control over their self-presentation does not mean that they can desist from this behavior. Indeed, the contrary is true; the deeper dissociation is utterly uncontrolled, and this makes it practically impossible for psychopaths to do anything else but con at the level of social valuations. Likewise, the same is true of the kind of rationalizations and trumped-up emotions psychopaths rely on. True, at this point, there is a level of conscious ego-involvement in these techniques, but it is a pathologically inflated ego we are talking about here, an ego that has lost the ability to produce either genuine reasons or genuine feelings. The psychopath's grandiosity may take him in, but it ought not take us in. He has lost the ability not to con people; he is a slave to this behavior. What appears to be the ultimate freedom is actually bondage.

The author was recently consulted by an actor who was about to undertake the role of a psychopath in a movie. As the various constituent elements of the disorder were explained in terms of thrill-seeking, grandiosity, and dissociation, the actor remarked with some justice that his own craft met this description. While on stage, he pointed out, he enjoyed the thrill of the occasion, he deliberately sought to command attention, and he called upon his own dissociative capacity in order to throw himself into his role.

The difference is that actors can control all three elements: They can confine their thrill-seeking to the hours between 7:30 and 10:00 in the evening plus two matinees during the week; they know there are times when they must yield the spotlight to their fellow actors lest they upstage them; and most important of all, they know deep down that they are not this or that English king and will soon have to catch a taxi back to a less-than-grand loft in Soho In order to make the distinction clear to the actor, the author fell back on James Joyce's well-known consultation with Carl Jung with regard to Joyce's schizophrenically ill daughter. Jung explained the loosening of associations characteristic of the disease, to which Joyce replied that this was precisely what he did in his writing. Jung answered, "Yes, but you are swimming in it; your daughter is drowning."

The psychopath, in short, cannot turn off the dissociative tendency. This sometimes wreaks diagnostic havoc in courtroom proceedings. During the trial of Bianchi, the defense brought forth evidence suggesting that he was a multiple personality and that crimes of the Hillside Strangler were done by a second self outside of Bianchi's control. In support of this contention, evidence derived from the use of hypnosis was also brought forth. In a celebrated battle of rival experts, Martin Orne won the case for the prosecution by arguing that Bianchi had faked being a multiple personality—the police searching his home found numerous psychological texts that might have helped Bianchi do this—and that he had faked hypnosis as well. With regard to the outcome, there can be little quarrel with Orne's strategy, but in our view he might have gone much further. For Bianchi was not just a malingerer; he was also faking being normal, faking consulting with his defense attorney, and faking under cross-examination. This man could only con people; there existed no counterpole of an inwardly valid set of truths that would allow one to admit to faking one thing and not everything else.

When dissociation runs riot in this fashion, the clinician is entitled to ask why these people do not "have the common decency to go crazy." Indeed, Cleckley originally supposed that they were crazy; in the 1941 edition of *The Mask of Sanity*, he suggested that psychopathy constituted a subtype of schizophrenia. By the late 1970s, however, he had amended that view in favor of the more modest claim that psychopathy was closer to psychosis than to neurosis in terms of the severity of the disorder. It is interesting to speculate how and why psychopaths avoid frank psychosis. Sullivan[25] has made the provocative observation that certain spontaneously remitting schizophrenics temporarily or permanently acquire certain psychopathic traits. The implication is that psychopathic traits somehow constitute an alternative to overt schizophrenic confusion. But true psychopaths seem never to have been crazy; it is as though their personality style grants them immunity in most social milieus against frankly psychotic developments.

Is it possible to drive a psychopath crazy?[26] Severe environmental deprivation, such as results from being put in solitary confinement within a prison, has been known to produce psychotic states both in psychopaths and in ordinary criminals. But here, too, psychopaths can be distinguished. When ordinary inmates develop a psychosis in this fashion, it acquires a momentum of its own and treatment is needed to bring them out of it. Psychopaths, by contrast, need only to be placed back into the prison milieu; once they are allowed to resume their typical pattern of acting out, their psychosis spontaneously remits. It would appear from this that schizophrenia represents a miscarriage of psychological processes that are developmentally and socially more complex than those of the psychopath. Schizophrenics have lost in their battle to establish a basic kernel of self. Psychopaths, by contrast, are not concerned with establishing a self; they are concerned only with maintaining an optimal level of stimulation coupled with an optimal opportunity for acting out. In etiological terms, our suspicion is that on a neglect–pampering continuum, the psychopath is more likely to come from a milieu loaded on the neglect end, the schizophrenic from the pampered end.[27] But what precisely constitutes the etiologically significant kinds of neglect in the case of the psychopath, we cannot say.

With the mention of etiologically significant variables, we feel obliged to pause for an observation with regard to diagnostic classifications and their relation to process taxonomies. Too frequently clinicians, when asked to make predictions about dangerousness, consult the literature on topics like dangerousness and violence, only to be confronted with a hodgepodge of observations derived from a mixed population. Some psychopaths are violent; so too, are some career criminals; so too, are some epileptics; so too, are some drug users; so too, are some schizophrenics; and so forth. The problem one so often encounters in the literature is that attributes of different logical types are combined willy-nilly. *Violence* is a behavioral unit; *drug abuser* is both a behavioral description and a rudimentary character portrait; *Psychopath* is at a higher logical level still. It denotes a recognizable personality syndrome that may or may not exhibit violent or drug-taking behaviors. In this context, our own suspicion is that the level of violence exhibited by any given psychopath will be highly correlated with the amount of overt physical abuse suffered in childhood as well as with the level of violence characteristic of the psychopath's immediate social milieu. But we would not necessarily expect these same correlations to obtain invariably for other clinical groups.

That last example may seem straightforward but the problem is more general still. If we hope to make progress in understanding the psychopath, we must understand which psychological processes are essential to the syndrome and which are peripheral. And in teasing out the etiology of the essential processes, we must be willing to cut across the walls of established diagnostic entities to observe whether or not the same or similar psychological factors obtain for any particular process, regardless of diagnostic designation. Take the issue of dissociation. It is clear that a profound reliance on dissociation is an essential hallmark of the psychopathic disorder. (Indeed, we would argue that together with an abnormally high psychological threshold of stimulation manifest in thrill-seeking and a profoundly disturbed relation to issues of power and dominance, dissociation constitutes part of the distinguishing triad of traits basic to this syndrome.) But when we compare the degree and quality of dissociative processes in the psychopath with the degree and quality of the same processes in other syndromes, do we arrive at generally valid psychological principles? Do we learn anything about etiologically significant environmental variables?[28] These are questions worth pursuing.[9] There is some evidence to suggest that the dissociation typical of multiple personality originates in the context of severe physical or sexual abuse in childhood. It is also clear that in some cases psychopathy arises from home situations. Nonetheless, it is likewise clear that the psychopathy syndrome, though it overlaps with multiple personality in respect to dissociation as a constituent mechanism, constitutes an inherently different response of the developing personality. Thus, we may ask what other factors besides physical or sexual abuse must be present to produce the particular outcome of psychopathic dissociation. In the multiple egos of developing children who have not yet left the magical stage, and thus are readily prepared to imagine themselves as more than one person, we have the grass-roots level of dissociative capacity. Faced with traumatic physical or sexual abuse, children at this stage readily defend themselves with the thought that the abuse happened to someone else; this imagined someone else then becomes the nucleus of a second personality. Children who have a high innate dissociative capacity do this readily; children with a low innate capacity have to work at it. It seems likely, therefore, that traumatic physical or sexual abuse is instrumental in heightening the child's capacity for and reliance on the mechanism of dissociation. What has to happen in psychopathic development, however, is for this heightened capacity to attach itself to the child's own antisocial behavior; currently, it is not clear how this comes about. It is quite possible that the link to antisocial behavior occurs somewhat later in childhood and that differential associative networks of the sort Sutherland described play an instrumental role.

Here let us observe that psychopaths have significant social relationships, relationships that are important in the maintenance of the disorder. Fritz Redl and David Wineman[29] discovered this to their chagrin when they set up a residential facility for antisocial youths. As they report in *Children Who Hate*, they were initially surprised and pleased to see their charges banding together into tight-knit groups until they discovered that the group functioned as a means of perpetuating pathology and resisting the demands of the therapeutic milieu. Redl and Wineman report in vivid clinical detail how the children were masters at using the group as a means of maintaining their essential ego deficits. The same reliance on interpersonal relations can also be seen in adult psychopaths, even in the most profoundly disturbed. Thus, in a majority of cases, serial killers are found to have employed the devices of an accomplice. And when they can be made to confess to the accomplice's existence, they invariably turn the tables on the accomplice, who not only killed, but mutilated the corpse, they say, and is really sick. In this way, they excuse their own behavior by dispersing its significance onto others. The serial killer Henry Lee Lucas, for example, decried his accomplice's alleged cannibalism. The accomplice, like the juvenile gang, protects psychopaths from a confrontation with their deficits through differential association. In this way, the innate dissociative capacity becomes more closely linked with antisocial trends.

This, then, in large overview is our portrait of the psychopath. The essential psychological mechanisms appear to be thrill-seeking, dissociation, and a profound disturbance in the relationship to issues of power and dominance manifested in a grandiose delusional belief in the exceptional nature of the self. Of these three traits, dissociation in all its myriad forms—psychopathic glibness, absence of guilt, semantic dementia—is the most readily observable, but all three are necessary to constitute the syndrome. (Obviously they interact. Dissociative mechanisms subserve both thrill-seeking and grandiosity. By the same token grandiosity becomes a rationale for thrill-seeking and an organizer of dissociative mechanisms. The techniques of rationalization rely on the dissociation of affect and the concomitant semantic dementia; so too does the absence of guilt. And so forth.) In the exercise of these psychological mechanisms, moreover, psychopaths rely on select interpersonal relations as both social insulators and preferred social instigators to further psychopathy.

Clearly, we are dealing with something that both goes beyond the exigencies of intergroup competition and is qualitatively different in some respects from the special case Lifton has described. The phenomenon is quite unusual. We seem to be dealing with an apparently far-reaching if largely covert decline in values that tends to become manifest in individual behavior with the individual's ascension to a position of power. This phenomenon in the individual is mirrored in and complemented by the public perception of it as expectable and implicitly acceptable. Values have lost their compelling quality in certain circumstances and everyone knows about it. This malignant phenomenon of normalized psychopathy in positions of power,[30] like the more benign psychopathy of ordinary life that it is heir to, must derive from certain peculiarities of our ordinary social relationships. It is to these that I now turn.

3

War and Social Distress

Images of the Enemy

> Events are in the saddle and ride
> mankind.
> Ralph Waldo Emerson

> Modern journalism justifies its own
> existence by the great Darwininan
> principle of the survival of the
> vulgarist.
> Oscar Wilde, *The Critic as an Artist*

Though it is possible to think of war in terms of purely objective aims, as the continuation of diplomacy by other means, as Clausewitz's famous phrase has it, "War is inconceivable without a clearly defined image of the enemy." States at war may justify their strategic interests with rationales derived from current social and historical conditions. But the sheer aggressiveness of war, the use of unlimited force in the pursuit of those strategic objectives, both requires and engenders a deep-seated sense of enmity between participants. A battlefield without enemies cannot exist.[1]

What is true for battlefields readily becomes true for whole societies through emotional contagion. This is especially true in the modern age, when the exigencies of industrialized warfare require mass mobilization on a national scale and when, as a result, civilian populations are regularly targeted for destruction as an indispensable military resource. War is no longer the preoccupation of the professional soldier; civilian populations must be prepared both to suffer devastation and to tolerate having their own armies inflict equivalent devastation on their equally unarmed counterparts. To

59

make that stance psychologically tolerable, and even more, to make it compelling, an agreed-upon image of the enemy must gain widespread currency. Defining an image of the "enemy" on a mass scale of enmification is the psychological prerequisite for modern warfare.

What is true for modern warfare in general is even more applicable to the logic of conflict in the nuclear age. The awesome, uncontrollable destructive capacity of nuclear weapons makes them of almost no value in a battlefield situation: Blast and radiation rain on the just and the unjust alike. The real value of nuclear weapons, well evidenced by their only actual use in a conflict, lies in their ability to wreak catastrophic damage on civilian populations.

Because of their uncontrollable destructiveness, the only logical target of nuclear weapons is the homeland of the other combatant. And because of the predictably catastrophic result of such use, the decision to use them transcends ordinary military logic. Genocide is by no means new—the ancient Assyrians piled high the bones of their victims to make small mountains—but only in the nuclear age has genocide become a routine military contingency. And just as the contemporary military planner must embrace genocide as his strategy of last resort, so he must live with the counterthreat that the same catastrophe will be unleashed against his own population. Genocide is now a fact of life for the strategist. Indeed, the only relevant question from a strategic standpoint is whether it might be possible, through first use, to lay waste the opposing country before it has a chance to respond.

We are all familiar with the doctrine of mutual assured destruction, or MAD. As long as each nuclear power retains enough weapons to annihilate the population of the other, even after a first strike against its own weapons, then the decision to initiate a nuclear exchange becomes irrational. In the language of arms control, the protection of weapons is morally good, while the protection of populations is morally bad. The premise was explained to Soviet Prime Minister Kosygin by Secretary of Defense McNamara during the administration of Lyndon Johnson. So long as populations go undefended, while weapons are sufficiently protected to survive a surprise attack, then each nuclear power holds the civilian population of the other hostage and a condition of mutual deterrence necessarily obtains. War will not occur.

Yet if widespread "enmification" during peacetime is indeed the single most salient feature of our current civilization, it is one that goes largely undiscussed in the literature of the social sciences. It is as though it were too pervasive to draw comment. Like fish in the ocean, all we know is water, so it doesn't occur to us to take notice of it. Indeed, until very recently, well over half the population of this country had never known any other reality than this—that the Russians are our enemy and that we must prepare to destroy them since they are preparing to destroy us. The nuclear age has thus brought to a culmination a trend that has steadily been gaining momentum during the nineteenth and twentieth centuries: the employment of images of the enemy on a collective scale as a way of enlisting mass mobilization for purposes of war. Such are the emotional exigencies of imagined nuclear genocide that such collective enmity has become a permanent feature of "peace."

"Enmification" is a process that goes beyond objective and historical conditions. It entails psychological processes that run very deep and that rapidly acquire their own momentum. Having an "enemy" goes far deeper than merely having a competitor or an adversary. To have an "enemy" is in a sense to be possessed. One no longer feels entirely in command of one's own destiny: there is an enemy out there, and one's own fate is tied to his. And not only does one feel out of control, in an important psychological sense, one truly is out of control. Ultimately, the enemy comes to dominate one's thoughts and feelings to the point where one is virtually bewitched by that combination of fear and hatred that Nietzche defined as the "absence of peace of mind." In this sense, the enemy comes to be projected as a malevolent kind of "shadow" self.

In human iconography, having a shadow is the symbol *par excellence* for man's mysterious innerness, for his possession of moral and psychological qualities that are not readily visible to the outside world. In this vein, we should note that in folklore it is a hallmark of the devil that he casts no shadow. But by the same token, when man confronts the Other, especially when the Other hails from a different culture, he is led to question what lies concealed inside. And now the shadow readily becomes concretized and projected— it is given malevolent substance in the personification of the enemy. "Enmification" is a basic human tendency, as much a part of our potential as are our loftiest ideals; but as with all our tendencies, it can readily yield pathological results under certain conditions. However, the fact that it is such a basic tendency and is so deeply embedded within us makes it all the harder to observe rationally. Thus, in addition to the cultural blinders, both intended and inadvertent, that the possibility of a nuclear accident has imposed on American society, we must also contend with the fundamental elusiveness of the process of enmification: to separate what is truly substance from what is mere shadow is no simple task.

Approaches to the Psychology of "Enmification"

While we have become accustomed to think in terms of national enemies, the truth is that a nation cannot hate, only its citizens can. When we speak of collective enmity, then, we are talking about a social-psychological process that exists on multiple levels. As soon as we begin to talk about the "Soviet threat" or "international communism," our thinking tends to collapse the individual and the collective levels. Again, as De Gaulle noted, a nation does not have friends; it has only interests. And if a nation cannot have friends, in an important sense it cannot have enemies either, but only adversaries and competitors who oppose its interests.

This is more than mere semantics. Enmity is a visceral, powerfully felt phenomenon that can only be truly meaningful on an individual level. Collective enmity entails marshaling this phenomenon and redirecting it at targets often far removed from the individual's own experience. Sometimes the process breaks down and reveals its inherent dubiousness, as when Muhammad Ali refused to be inducted into the military service saying, "I got nothing against them Vietcongs." Indeed, in the early 1960s very few Americans had anything against the Vietcong. What is remarkable is that many of them somehow thought they did, and could be induced to go off to war on that basis.

Marshaling public opinion around any given image of the enemy entails complex social processes operating in conjunction with the psychology of the individual. Living in an age that takes mass wartime mobilization for granted, we have become accustomed to it, but we do well to remember that collective "enmification" is not always rational.

What we seek, then, is an understanding of "enmification" as a process which, while it has profound roots in the individual psyche, can in some situations be manipulated for purposes of mass mobilization. One way to approach the issue is to think in terms of the psychological utility of identifying an enemy. When an individual is under great stress, particularly the kind of stress that arises from social disorder, this is felt as diffuse anxiety. There arises a sense of being threatened, but it is a vague, undifferentiated threat, at least initially. Having a clear-cut enemy is obviously preferable — one can channel one's emotional energies—much in the way that anger or even a well-focused fear is preferable to a diffuse sense of panic. And so even the best of us at times resorts to the creation of a personal bogeyman, someone whom we can all hate, and feel better about it.

In some ways, the function of ideologies is to organize individual antipathies along collective lines. Not only is there comfort in numbers, but there is also the possibility of organizing an effective group response. The logic of group action intertwines with the emotional needs of the individual under stress to produce a shared image of the enemy. Such is the power of the emotional dynamic, however, that the process easily slides into irrationality. From an emotional standpoint, it is often much easier to wage war than to cope with the frustrations of peacetime. And when the organs of propaganda come into play via the mass media, the potential for irrationality grows immeasurably. A chasm opens up between the need for effective adaptation and the need for emotional closure as individual antipathies become collectively redirected against this or that national enemy. Surprisingly, many, many individuals find the overall result emotionally satisfying.

It cannot be said that the pioneers in dynamic psychology left behind a well worked out theory of how "enmification" works on either an individual or a collective basis; but if we survey their disparate contributions, we can hope to make a start on the problem. Perhaps the best place to begin is with Adler, who in his own life maintained an active participation in Socialist politics and always sought to cast his theories in a social perspective. Adler's basic contribution to the psychology of war is the idea that it derives from an absence of community feeling, a view he is said to have come to while pondering war's ravages from the safety of a Viennese cafe.

The thrust of Adler's notion amounts to a correction of his previous theory—elaborated in various versions during the years immediately after his collaboration with Freud ended—that neurotic mechanisms could best be understood through their social dimensions. Viewed in this light, neurotics sought various social gains, while safeguarding their own weaknesses, through a variety of unconscious tricks by which they hoodwinked both themselves and others. This is clearly a teleological perspective—the neurotic is aiming toward something—and in *The Neurotic Constitution*[2] Adler elevated this aspect of his paradigm above all others. In that revised view, Adler argued that all men aim at realizing certain personal fictions ("guiding images" might be a better term) in the conduct of their lives, and that the neurotic was chiefly distinguished by the asocial quality of the personal fiction that had been adopted. Whereas another individual might wish to be a father, or a judge, the neurotic wanted to be a king, or queen, and thus be catered to in matters large and small. The neurotic does not consciously know this, of course—that would spoil it—but only feels the resentment, anxiety, and hostility that result from every contact with a social reality that fails to confirm the guiding image. These feelings, in turn, become the raw material for the neurotic's career as a sufferer by which he seeks to achieve the same degree of personal elevation through other means.

The difficulty with this view, useful though it may be as a clinical heuristic, is that it fails to capture something essential about normal psychology. All of us operate on the basis of some guiding image, even if we do push it to the neurotic extreme. The notion of community feeling amounts to an attempt to capture that missing ingredient; in essence, the idea is that healthy individuals can orient themselves toward the needs and ideals of their fellow citizens and use these to shape their own guiding images. The general absence of such community feeling, further, is one of the prerequisites for the psychology of domination and hate that characterizes belligerents in wartime. Put simply, the enemy is the person toward whom one has no social feeling. Neurotics acquire enemies easily because they lack social feeling. Nations acquire enemies on much the same basis. What is needed to cure both war and neurosis is the same.

The basic problem with Adler's overall approach has since become obvious: It rests too heavily on the general Socialist belief that domestic social conditions, with their warping effect on the psychology of the individual, are the sole and sufficient cause of international conflict. The historical irony is that it was the very war during which Adler came up with his view that first proved the fundamental fallacy of this part of the Socialist plank: during the First World War, Socialists all over Europe enlisted in the military machines of their respective countries. The capacity for social feeling, as the Spartans knew, was no obstacle to war—or to having enemies. In general, Adler's theory suffers from a failure to distinguish different levels of analysis; it invokes the social dimension, but only insofar as it impacts on the psychology of the individual. It thus forfeits any chance to distinguish between processes that can only be understood in terms of the organization of society and those that can properly be attributed to individual development.

Freud had even less to say about the phenomenon of "enmification" attending the Great War. To be sure, he wrote an interesting essay on the general euphoria of war in which he highlighted the role of death, the argument being that as death became commonplace, the sense of risk returned to life, making it seem more worth living. But Freud had little to say about the psychology of having an enemy and personally he took what amounted to a rooting interest in the progress of the hostilities. (While the fact has not generally drawn comment, it was made a precondition for relaunching the international psychoanalytic movement after the war that the principals agree *not* to discuss what they had just lived through.)

It is sometimes said that the war did impact on Freud's theory in one respect: It led to his subsequent espousal of a "death instinct" whose most frequent manifestation was its outward-turned forms of destructiveness. Certainly later in life Freud became increasingly sensitized to the role of destructiveness in human affairs, both in his theories and, tragically, in his own social milieu. But the theory of the "death instinct" in Freud's rendition sheds no additional light on what is involved in destructiveness. Nor can it be said that Melanie Klein's subsequent (and brilliant) elaborations of that theory surpass the master's in that regard. For at bottom, all that is being discussed are the mechanisms by which an inborn capacity to hate is directed during the infant's development. Intuitively we know that people are born with a capacity to hate, but this tells us little about what is entailed in the social psychology of "enmification" in the adult.

Somewhat more useful in regard to the general idea of a "death instinct" is its reinterpretation as proposed by Erich Fromm in the middle of his career. Fromm[3] proposed that an urge to die arose from what he called "negative transcendence." Where the individual could not find meaning in his life, indeed where he no longer even sought such meaning, then the capacity for transcendence that is inherent to mankind turned into a malevolent psychological force that sought death and that could readily be turned outward as a sadistic destructiveness. Certainly, such an evil psychological turn could everywhere be detected in the phenomenon of Nazism, with which Fromm was familiar, just as it can today be found (in somewhat different form) among a certain subgroup of psychopaths.

The problem with this line of argument is that it relies too heavily on a pathological model. "Enmification" is far too general a phenomenon to be explained solely by reference to this or that clinical entity. Negative transcendence may indeed explain much about the psychology of certain virulent hatemongers who may form the vanguard in national campaigns of "enmification." But it fails to tell why their message should be accepted by a populace, nor is it informative as to the structure of the mechanism of dissemination.

Of all the pioneering depth psychologists, Jung perhaps deserves the most credit for plainly grasping the significance of the social dimension in "enmification." Having an "enemy" in Jung's terms is a general "collective" phenomenon, and that is the first fact that must be observed about it. Riding out the First World War in neutral Switzerland, Jung was in a unique position to retain an empirical perspective and, to his credit, he availed himself of it. The following was penned in December 1916[4]:

> The psychological concomitants of the present war—above all, the incredible brutalization of public opinion, the mutual slanderings, the unprecedented fury of destruction, the monstrous flood of lies, and man's incapacity to call a halt to the blood demon—are uniquely fitted to force upon the attention of every thinking person the problem of the chaotic unconscious which slumbers easily beneath the ordered world of consciousness. This war has pitilessly revealed to civilized man that he is still a barbarian, and has at the same time shown what an iron scourge lies in store for him if ever again he should be tempted to make his neighbor responsible for his own evil qualities. (p. 4)

In trying to explicate what he meant by making one's neighbor responsible for one's own evil qualities, Jung went on to propose a pair of universal human structures that worked in tandem with one another. The first involved a tendency to identify too readily with one's various social roles, and most especially to claim for oneself the various virtues that are typically ascribed to those roles. That tendency Jung labeled the "persona." The second, reciprocal tendency Jung labeled the "shadow." It consists of all those inclinations that do not fit the image of the persona and are thus suppressed— and projected. In the romantic literature of the nineteenth century, such a projection was often represented as a *doppelganger*, an evil, pursuing double, and Jung regularly illustrated his idea of the shadow with examples taken from this genre. But as the passage quoted above makes clear, Jung also realized that the same basic process was readily discernible in the wartime psychology of defining the enemy.

What Jung took for granted at the time, even if he took no great pains to spell it out, was that the link from establishing an enemy on an individual basis to establishing one collectively was readily supplied by processes of emotional contagion. It was then generally held that such emotional contagion was inherent in man as a species, and that it underlay both the psychology of suggestion and of concerted group action. The theory was perhaps best expounded by Wilfred Trotter[5] in his remarkable, if now neglected, work, *The Herd Instinct in Times of Peace and War*. It was partially in response to Trotter's work, also to Jung's and Adler's, that in the early 1920s Freud himself turned to the analysis of what in German is called *massenpsychologie*. In essence, Freud sought to reinterpret the processes of emotional contagion in terms of the centrality of the Oedipus complex. What was key in his view was the common identification with the leader of the group, himself a substitute for the father; this common identification both linked members of the group with one another and formed the basis for the group identity as a whole. Aggression against the leader, the flip side of the original Oedipal ambivalence toward the father, became taboo and had to be discharged against outsiders.

The advantage of Freud's refinement was that it brought into focus the vertical dimension inherent in corrected group action. Contagion works well as an explanation for a riot, for a stock market panic; but purposeful and sustained group activity requires an organized hierarchy of command. That hierarchy, in turn, secures legitimization in part through emotional processes that touch deeply on the individual psyche.

If there is a weakness in Freud's view, it is that by appealing to the family, and even more to a universally inherited propensity of the psyche to view questions of authority in terms of the Oedipal complex, he arrived at a view of social structure that overestimated its stability. Both authority and the idealization that subserves it depend on a community consensus with regard to fundamental values; they depend, in other words, on a shared mythology or worldview. Where that consensus breaks down, the resemblance to the family is lost and Oedipal ties are no longer sufficient to insure social order. Jung may justly be said to have been sensitive to this aspect of the problem: in the 1930s, he came to argue that in periods of disorder, when the established myths of a society disintegrated, the stage was set for fresh eruptions of material from the collective unconscious, the "shadow" included. Though he can justly be accused of being inconstant to this point, Jung was keenly, if intermittently, aware of how destructive such eruptions might be as the worst of man's demons were set loose upon the world. The subsequent history of the twentieth century has confirmed the pessimistic side of his theory. (The optimistic side of Jung's view had it that such fresh eruptions of the collective unconscious had potentially creative, and evolutionary, significance. Recent history has not confirmed this part of the argument.)

But let us break off this survey here, recognizing that we have fallen well short of the mark. If there is a commonality in the various views so far discussed, it is to be found in the convergence around three points. First, enmification has to be understood as part and parcel of a process of self-inflation. Whether defined in terms of Adler's fictions, Jung's persona, or Freud's identification with the father, the inflated self wants to know only its virtues; its vices are relegated to some other world. There they readily form the raw material for projections onto the image of one's enemies, real or imagined. The end result is that one feels oneself to be the "hero," noble in all respects, who is called to do battle with an unspeakable foe. Second, this process is readily communicable through emotional contagion, whereas its contrary, self-reflection and transcendence, is not. For the former entails heightened emotional expressions with inherently powerful suggestive effect, whereas the latter can be achieved only through mature emotional development and individuation. Third, the internal organization of a society, its authority structures and its legitimizing myths, can exercise a decisive role in the process of the enmification. In general, the less coherent a society's values, and the less secure the position of its leadership, the more virulent its appeal to processes of enmification.

DISSOCIATION AND THE PSYCHOLOGY OF CONFLICT

From the foregoing it should strike us that the process of "enmification," in its pathological manifestations, exhibits a certain homology between the individual and the collective levels. In both areas, it is regularly associated with a loss of hierarchal integration and a concomitant decline in conscious, rational self-direction. We can say that the psychologically well-integrated individual is aware of his own vices; he does not need to invent enemies to project his own evils outside himself. Likewise, the well-integrated society can approach situations of conflict in a rational manner: It can promote and defend its interests without the distorting prism of imagining international bogeymen. Interestingly enough, though the kind of integration we are speaking of is clearly different on the individual level than it is on the collective, in conditions of breakdown they tend to meet and to converge. The poorly integrated individual is likely to become both more conformist and more subject to the emotional contagions of his group. Likewise, the poorly integrated society is likely to resort to the manipulation of emotional contagion on a mass scale to supply what is otherwise lacking, a sense of direction derived from shared values.

An alternative way of phrasing matters is to speak in terms of dissociation, broadly conceived as the counterbalancing tendency opposed to integration. Kurt Goldstein,[6] in his famous book *The Organism*, makes the pertinent point that despite the fundamental unity of the organism, certain processes within it have an inner organization of their own and in conditions of pathology can become functionally independent of the normal integrative processes. This is true for pathologies of the central nervous system and for social systems, as well as for individual psychopathology, where the parts of the integrated system of the personality can become wrenched free from the main system, resulting in varying degrees of abnormality in behavior.

Such an overall scheme is readily compatible with the work of Jean Piaget, who clearly demonstrated that a functional unity at the symbolic or ego level is achieved only over time and at a relatively slow pace, as the child moves from one gradually achieved level to the next in the process of development. One can perhaps best conceive the developing child in terms of behavioral manifestations that appear as if they were directed by multiple egos. This is quite reasonable, after all, for the child in its development literally has not determined who it is to be. Because dissociation is so intimately related to the breakdown of the integrative mechanisms of the mind, it is often confused with psychoanalytic concepts like repression and regression. But, by and large, dissociation can be thought of as potentially normal. In the healthy organism the dissociative processes are part and parcel of the overall capacity for selective adaption, just as in the individual they contribute to the ability to live in terms of different systems of values at different times.

What we are concerned with here is the specific circumstance when dissociative processes begin to outstrip the integrative processes, resulting in the functional autonomy of certain subprocesses. Specifically, we would like to advance the hypothesis that enmification represents a dissociative breakdown of the normal processes that regulate social conflict, both internally and externally. It can be taken as axiomatic that in any complex social system, conflict is inevitable and the capacity for aggression in the service of one's own values and prerogatives is indispensable. It can also be taken as axiomatic that the same capacity for aggression in one's adversaries necessarily raises the stakes in any conflict, a defenseless opponent being no opponent at all. Thus there exists, in any conflict situation, what Bateson[7] characterized as a symmetrical tendency toward escalation. Against this tendency, however, there usually are pitted countervailing processes between participants, processes that are asymmetrical or, in Bateson's terminology, complementary, that work to end conflict. Thus, for example, the aggressive behavior of one participant may tend to induce submissive behavior on the part of the other.

Plainly, for conflict resolution to occur, two things are necessary. First, the symmetrical and asymmetrical processes subsuming conflict must be sufficiently well balanced to avoid a behavioral runaway of the system. And second, the nature of this balance must be such that new learning can occur among participants during the course of the exchange. This new learning, in turn, can perhaps be conceptualized in terms of a reevaluation of perceptions in search of common assumptions with regard to both practice and outcome. This can be seen even on a simple level. For example, between two members of an animal species involved in mutual threat displays in the course of a territorial dispute, the nature of the learning is straightforward: as soon as it is mutually established between them which is the stronger, the weaker is allowed to quit the field, the inherent structure of the animal yielding an implicit value consensus that the stronger animal is entitled to it. In human conflict, of course, such an emergent value consensus must be mediated symbolically, but the basic structure stays the same. Likewise, in the animal, the interaction itself is regulated by inborn mechanisms that dictate the proper conduct of the struggle—it is not "cricket" for one elk simply to ambush another broadside. But in the human, the conduct of a conflict must again be mediated symbolically, i.e., in terms of mutually acceptable rules of what "playing fair" consists of.

The intervention of a symbolic layer in the regulation of human conflict deserves further comment. It is too often assumed that this is somehow a more tentative, and shaky, mode of existence, as compared with the more fundamental, and altogether more visceral, modes of behavior that represent the anlage of our species' animal past. Beneath the rational man of compromise and conciliation (the prejudice runs) lurks a demonic beast, and, between them, the beast is really the stronger. Much contemporary theorizing in both sociobiology and international relations unwittingly adopts just such a plank. The truth is, however, that we are really quite good at our special forte of mediating conflict symbolically—so good, in fact, that we indulge in it regularly just for the fun of exploring our abilities. For throughout history, men have always loved to invent and play games, which are nothing other than the creation of wholly arbitrary conflicts for the sheer delight of seeing them symbolically mediated. Moreover, even when the ordinary process of conflict resolution breaks down, what emerges is not any putative beast within—we pass over in silence the slander against animal psychology—but a process of *resymbolization*. It is important to realize that enmification, no less than the ordinary process of social conflict, involves man's highest capacities as a creature who relies on the symbolic mediation of its behavior.

In a different vein, it is also important to realize that the ordinary processes of social conflict may generate massive, even revolutionary, social change without enmification. While it may be true that the history of man is largely the history of warfare, and thus of enmification, it is not necessarily true that that is the only way to alter fundamentally the way societies operate. Gandhi and Martin Luther King, for example, were both able to alter profoundly the social structure of entire nations without resorting to processes of "enmification." For Gandhi, it wasn't the British people who opposed India's demand for independence (a cultural value the British understood and cherished). Rather, the problem lay in the inability on the part of the British administration to appreciate that Indians had learned and absorbed such a concept from their British stewards. Likewise, Dr. King avoided the process of enemy-making in that he did not accuse white Americans of racism, and then blame them for racial oppression, but instead argued that the values of the American way of life had to be applied to all in accordance with our basic concepts of freedom and equality. White Americans were not the problem; racism was. In both cases, there was a strong push for an underlying agreement on values, and an avoidance of the strategy of particularizing the opponents as enemies per se.

With "enmification," the reverse is true: The opponent is particularized and he is resymbolized to appear both implacable and menacing. He is menacing in that he is portrayed as representing a clear and dangerous threat to survival. And he is implacable in that he is held incapable of sharing in the fundamental value system of the protagonist. The result is that processes that subsume aggression become dissociated from the subsuming, and unless these parties can be effectively isolated from further contact, a runaway behavioral system necessarily results.

It would be comforting to suppose that "enmification" is always a pathological process, and indeed such a proposition, though unprovable, may be true. But the dangerous reality is that "enmification" can and does get loose in human affairs and, once it does, impinges on the peace-loving no less than on the warlike. Consider the revolutionary fervor of the Ayatollah Khomeini in his address on the anniversary of the prophet Mohammed's birthday in 1983:

> If one permits an infidel [a nonbeliever] to continue in his role as a corrupter of the earth, his moral suffering will be all the worse. If one kills the infidel, and this stops him from perpetrating his misdeeds, his death will be a blessing to him. For if he remains alive, he will become more and more corrupt. War is a blessing for the world and for all nations. It is God who incites men to fight and kill. The Koran says: "Fight until all corruption and all rebellion have ceased." The wars the Prophet led against all infidels were a blessing for all humanity.... [A] religion without war is an incomplete religion. If his holiness Jesus ... had been given more time to live, he would have acted as Moses did, and wielded the sword.

This man, by his own declaration, *is* an enemy—and proud of it. One could not confront him without at once suspecting that there was no basis for conciliation, nor any rules for playing fair. One tended immediately to be pulled into a symmetrical relationship with him.

But, we should notice the structure of the Ayatollah's argument. For essential to his portrait of the "infidel" is the element of dehumanization. This is the ultimate omega point for all forms of "enmification." A mental Rubicon is crossed in thinking about enemies. Where most cultures prescribe rewards for controlling violent emotions and behaviors, the process of enmification constitutes a resymbolizing process that heightens and nurtures angry and violent feelings. As Keen[8] put it, a "consensual paranoia" emerges in war-oriented societies. It is a pathological process that results finally in a delusional system of thought and feeling. From a religious angle, the enemy becomes nothing less than evil incarnate, a "fake person," an imposter, a malefactor pretending to be human. In more general terms, the enemy may be characterized as racially, linguistically, ethnically, or physically different, but the difference is invariably held to be both fundamental and noxious. From a psychological standpoint, the creation of an enemy entails a psychosocial "kenosis"—an emotional catharsis and outpouring of oneself in an unusual way; one's least desirable traits and dispositions are projected onto another, transferred to the enemy, so that the presence of the enemy means the dissolution of those unsavory characteristics that may have previously defined oneself.[9] One becomes more "human" as the enemy becomes less so.

Dehumanization involves two kindred but distinct processes. Self-directed dehumanization relates to intrapsychic events where the self protects itself by immunizing itself against stress-laden situations that threaten to be traumatizing. Self-directed dehumanization is not necessarily emotionally disabling, nor is it entirely dysfunctional. In many ways it is an integral part of everyday life where the individual must defuse emotionally explosive or painful facts by developing an equanimity, a sort of callousness that shields the individual against empathetic identification that may be wholly nonadaptive.

Self-dehumanization practiced selectively is characteristic of normal occupational routines among many professional groups in our highly bureaucratic social structure. In medicine and law enforcement, to mention just two fields, individuals must learn to detach themselves to some extent (an extent that is virtually impossible to routinize, let it be noted) from patients, clients, offenders, and victims if they are to perform their jobs efficiently and effectively. For those who interact with physicians and police, this studied reserve and emotional aloofness may appear as indifference—a lack of comforting and reassuring empathy.

Object dehumanization, the other side of self-dehumanization, describes the process and dynamics whereby the individual depersonalizes the other; enmification takes that process one step further and reduces the other to a "thing" that is potentially dangerous. Redl and his associates[10] describe the psychology of object dehumanization in terms of

> ... a defense against painful or overwhelming emotions [that] entails a decrease in a person's sense of his own individuality and in his perception of the humanness of other people. The misperceiving of others ranges from viewing them *en bloc* as "subhuman" or "bad human" (a long-familiar component of group prejudice) to viewing them as nonhuman as though they were inanimate items or dispensable supplies. As such, their maltreatment or even their destruction may be carried out or acquiesced in with relative freedom from restraints of conscience or feelings of brotherhood.

Some of the familiar psychological defenses making up dehumanization include repression, isolation of affect, and depersonalization. Combined they facilitate the evolution of the psychic structure that can tolerate mass murder in the context of violence and combat. This "tough-mindedness," as it were, transcends hatred, anger, and hysteria—the ordinary emotional tones we associate with the battlefield—and constitutes an emotional coarsening that renders those emotions superfluous. Perhaps the best (or worst) example of the psychological posture was that of Nazi death camp operators who closed themselves down to the massive and constant suffering and pain to which they were exposed everyday. But such a posture is also to be found in modern warfare, which can be fought in a sanitized fashion, waged almost by proxy through the use of intricate machines of great destructive capability. Enemies can be almost entirely depersonalized, reduced to little more than pins on a map or, as Lifton[11] has described electronic warfare in Vietnam, "blips on a screen."

Nonetheless, even in the era of technological war, it remains true militarily that only ground troops can take and hold land. And soldiers who must fight these campaigns necessarily have a "hands-on" relationship with the enemy and so must develop more emotionally virulent defenses against identifying with the humanity of their opponent. Thus, American soldiers who had some contact with the Japanese, Germans, North Koreans, Chinese, or Vietnamese constructed racial and ethnic stereotypes such as "gooks," "slopes," "krauts," or "chinks" that, at the cost of emotional impoverishment, made it easier for one soldier to destroy another, for the other was already diminished in his humanity.

Self- and object-directed dehumanization are inevitably heightened in situations where the threat of combat is present. And where the setting is strange, and the expectations unclear, the mixture of threat and confusion can produce murderous results, as in Vietnam. There, to the horror of the American public, American soldiers proved that they were capable of the worst sort of atrocities against civilians. But what was immediately palpable to people back home—that the victims of My Lai were women and children—was exactly what was absent from the point of view of the soldiers involved. From their point of view, they were merely enacting a due measure of revenge. Without a clear-cut enemy or a clear-cut battle-field to help organize perception, the processes of "enmification" and object dehumanization ran amok, as Lifton[12] notes:

> [T]he murderous behavior of the GI's [was] a direct result of the contradictions of their situation, which derives in turn from the illusory American cosmology.... Thrust into this alien revolution in an alien culture, assigned an elusive enemy who is everyone and no one, sent into dangerous nonbattles in a war lacking the most elementary rules or structures of meaning, what do we expect him to do? He in fact finds himself in exactly the situation Jean-Paul Sartre has described as inevitably genocidal—troops from an advanced industrial nation engaged in a counterinsurgency action in an underdeveloped area, against guerrillas who merge with the people. (pp. 40–41)

THE VITALITY OF HATE

There are two distinct processes by which the process of enmification can spread within a population. The first is through the ordinary means of cultural transmission. The human mind lives on images, absorbing and re-creating them as a basis for understanding and action. The agents of socialization—the family, the school, the peer group, and the media—guide our doings by providing the background stocks of knowledge and the cognitive maps that allow us to locate, perceive, identify, and label a seemingly infinite number of concrete occurrences. Generating new world pictures and new definitions and identities for others is basic to all social change. The force of the change depends on the degree to which symbolizing agencies (those that produce a society's ideology) manage to saturate what Goffman[13] calls the primary frameworks that organize experience with new or reformed visions and ideas about others. But these frameworks that regulate the conduits between the individual and the world are pliable; they can and have been duped, coaxed, and regularly manipulated by individuals for purposes other than the transmission of cultural values. The significance of "enmification" is that it brings into play an essentially paranoid system that deputizes new and pathological symbols to represent reality. Those identified as enemies occupy a specific position in these systems, a position that is fashioned to evoke responses that dehumanize.

The advantage, if one can call it that, of "enmification" is that it fosters self-deception in the service of promoting action. The expansion of America across the continent to the Pacific Ocean may have been historically inevitable, but it was morally embarrassing insofar as it was recognized that the Indians who heretofore lived on the land had prior claim to it. The moral problem disappeared once the red man was turned into an enemy, into a dumb (but potentially dangerous) savage. Similarly, the coordination of law enforcement on a national scale became a practical necessity with the improvement of the national system of transportation, most especially with the improvement of roads and the simultaneous mass production of automobiles. Once the criminal became mobile, and able to cross state lines quickly and at his own whim, law enforcement agents had to do the same. It more or less naturally fell to agents of the federal government to be the ones to do this. But extending federal authority in this way raised serious problems with regard to legal autonomy of the individual states. Not only did such an expansion of federal power conflict with cherished notions of states' rights, but it also raised the specter of conflicting jurisdictions and the possibility that federal law would come to supersede local law in other, noncriminal matters. In short, it was not such a simple matter as the practical problem of catching criminals seemed to suggest. But the larger issues were readily bypassed once J. Edgar Hoover hit on the public relations ploy by bringing out a list of "public enemies," each with his own numerical rank in the hierarchy of infamy.

The idea of "public enemies" is intrusive. Obviously, each of the criminals so identified was indeed a dangerous person, someone whose apprehension and incarceration was devoutly to be desired. But to what degree can they be thought to be enemies of "the public"? Surely, they were less of a threat to the overall populace than any number of other threats arising from the social and economic conditions of the time. But unlike poverty, say, or disease, this threat could be particularized and individualized. Therein lay the popularity of the "public enemies" concept and its effectiveness. Incidentally, the strategy is not new: Foucault[14] has described the grizzly torture and ultimate dismemberment that befell one Damiens, an eighteenth-century regicide. Through the bizarre iconography of his torture, death, and burial without sacraments, Damiens's act was defined as a blasphemy against the divinely established monarchical order. For his breach in the cosmically divined reality, Damiens paid with more than his life. The sacrifice of this particular "enemy" became, in effect, an inverted, paranoid sacrament meant to restore a social policy that felt itself violated. The ultimate rationality of that order, meanwhile, was thereby left unquestioned.

This, then, is the logic of declaring public enemies. By particularizing certain individuals as a threat to the established social order, ultimately to civilization, a society gains license to perpetuate that order without further reflection on it. Debate ceases, the hour for discussion is past, and action begins. There are clearly times in human affairs—Churchill jumps to mind—when just such a step is called for. But, by the same token, there are also clearly times when such a step is not called for. And at these times, enmification readily substitutes for public discussion. Noam Chomsky has made the interesting point that the Iran-Contra scandal arose not because of public indifference but precisely because a great many watchdog groups were intensely involved in this area of foreign policy and had succeeded in mobilizing public opinion about it. What then happened, in Chomsky's felicitous phrase, was that the *people* became the supposed "enemy." The government decided that this new enemy had to be opposed, or rather duped, and took its own operations "off the books." Again, this kind of inverted enemy-making is scarcely new—it was plainly described by Ibsen in his famous drama, *Enemy of the People*—but the means for fostering it on a mass scale have been steadily increasing in modern times.

There is a second means whereby "enmification" may spread through a population, one that is all the more insidious for its seeming rationality. Here we have in mind "enmification" as a response to enmification in the other. Consider again the Ayatollah and how we so readily feel ourselves pulled into a symmetrical relationship with him. Insofar as he has declared us the enemy, we felt nothing more complicated than honorable self-defense. But it is more complicated, or at least it readily becomes so. Imagine the general hoopla that would result in the American media if a CIA assassination team sent the Ayatollah prematurely to his eternal reward. Or better yet, rather than imagine that event, the reader should merely recall the general self-congratulatory euphoria that followed in the wake of the bombing raid on Libya as well as more recently Baghdad. For the majority of the American population, the only thing to be regretted about that act of war, which was essentially a sneak attack against civilian targets, was that it failed to kill both Khadafy and Hussein.

But in what sense is either the Ayatollah, Khadafy, or Hussein different from us? If we take pride in a bombing raid that killed two of his children, then how should we expect Hussein or Khadafy to regard us? At this point, many Americans will be tempted to respond with the words that children so often use: "But *he* started it!" Moreover, it will be quickly brought up that Khadafy or Hussein is a terrorist, that he doesn't "play fair," and that therefore he doesn't deserve to be treated fairly either. But what all of this adds up to is that we feel ourselves entitled to do unto him what he has done unto us. We have become more like him, not less, as the process of enemy-making spreads to our own society.

In this sense, "enmification" can be compared to a virus, one that spreads from one society to the next through contact. If, as the phrase has it, a virus is trouble wrapped in a protein, then "enmification" is trouble wrapped up in the symbols of life, liberty, and self-defense. But surely some reader will want to respond that thinking about "enmification" in this fashion leads to pacifism, and ultimately to defenselessness. Not necessarily. The great Russian general of the Napoleonic era, Katusov, clearly recognized who his enemy was. But after the battle of Borodino, he just as plainly recognized that this enemy was so dangerous that he could not afford to engage him again in battle; he could not risk what was left of his army. Thus, while all of the officers under him urged again and again a new battle, Katusov waited, and waited, and won. The reality of the Russian winter was on his side; the compelling emotional logic of rushing to fight a hated enemy was not.

Katusov's example has general applicability. Granted that enemies may indeed exist, both in one's personal life and in international relations, one perforce must take some stance about how to deal with them. But often as not, the best course of action is to view them warily, while giving them a wide berth; the less interaction one has with an enemy, the less opportunity there is to suffer harm, and the less likely one is to be drawn into an escalating reciprocal struggle. As regards personal matters, the virtues of such a strategy are obvious. Indeed, one of the hallmarks of paranoid reactions is the failure to observe the simple rule. In paranoid reactions, the individual becomes completely dominated by a preoccupation with enemies, real and imagined; every aspect of life comes to be intimately related to the struggle, until finally the paranoid person gives the impression that he or she literally has no other reason to live. This, in fact, is the case at the clinical extremes: Deprive a paranoid schizophrenic of his persecutory object, and he or she rapidly falls into confusion.

But if the strategy of wary avoidance can be employed effectively in personal matters, surely it is out of place in international relations. After all, we live in an age of complex international interdependency, and it appears that there is no way to escape various confrontations around the globe. In such a context, wary avoidance rapidly gives way to isolationism, the dangers of which are well known, or so the argument goes. Here let us counter, first of all, that isolationism is as American as cherry pie. Indeed, early in our nation's history, it was the cornerstone of American foreign policy— "No Foreign War!"—and it is only in this century that the opposite prejudice has come to prevail. Moreover, as with any strategy, there exists a range of possible implementations. The chief danger with regard to a truly thoroughgoing isolationism would be economic. If we cut ourselves off from world markets, we will suffer. But it is not this danger that springs most rapidly to mind for most people. No; what they imagine is that by withdrawing from armed conflict in this or that area of the world, we will let this or that enemy prevail. In the long run, the thinking goes, our enemies will only grow stronger and in the ultimate confrontation we will pay dearly for not taking up the struggle sooner. This seemingly "tough-minded" preference for engagement, for interventionism rather than isolationism, has still come to form part of the prevailing consensus in contemporary political life. Its historical roots are relatively recent in origin, however, and it is to these that we now turn.

THE NAZI THREAT AND THE AMERICAN SOCIAL DREAM

Interventionism became a permanent part of American foreign policy during the course of the Second World War. Prior to that time, isolationism still held the upper hand, though popular enthusiasm

could be whipped up for the occasional military contest, whether
with Spain or Mexico or whomever, so long as it was quick and one-
sided. To be sure, the First World War was scarcely one-sided, and it
clearly engendered great enthusiasm; but let us recall that it had
been billed as "the war to end all wars" and that it was thought that
the "boys" would be home in time for Christmas. In short, though
Americans were willing to intervene internationally, they did so
with the presumption that it would all be over quickly and they
could go back to the satisfaction of peacetime. So much was this part
of the national consensus that years later the Franklin D. Roosevelt
administration, convinced that a long and costly war was inevitable,
had to whip up public sentiment in the last two years prior to the
attack on Pearl Harbor. (It has been suggested, in fact, that one
reason why the administration was so relatively unprepared for war
with Japan was that it was too busy trying to sell the prospect of war
with Germany.)

In historical retrospect, the Nazis made almost ideal enemies.
They were indeed dangerous, implacable, and evil. Moreover, in
their case, wary avoidance simply would not work, as first the
British and then the Russians discovered too late. They had to be
fought; moreover, they had to be annihilated. But if the Nazis were
the perfect enemy, the horror of whose deeds became only more
clearly substantiated after the war, we should pause to consider
their case all the more carefully lest we draw the wrong historical
conclusion.

To begin with, we must note that Germany had not always been
either powerful or militaristic. Indeed, until the forced unification
brought about under Prussian domination in 1870, Germany had
been no more than a collection of independent principalities, each
with its own separate foreign policy and incapable of coordinating a
common cause, except under the direst threats from without. In the
political cartoon of the early nineteenth century, Germany was
usually depicted as a callow youth dressed in a nightshirt and
holding a candle—"Sleepy Michel"—who invariably arrived too
late in international disputes to make a difference. Bismarck and his
successors changed that, of course, but whereas Bismarck himself
pursued a most careful foreign policy based on maintaining protective alliances above all, his successors mistook his belligerent posturing for the essence of his policy and ultimately led the nation into

the catastrophe of the First World War. When Germany's defeat and subsequent humiliation at the negotiating table was followed by the Great Depression, German political authority was bankrupt.

During the long years of political fragmentation prior to Bismarck, German aspirations had predictably focused on the issues of race and culture. If they were not yet a nation, the Germans could claim to be a *Volk*. In the crisis years of the 1930s, this claim to folkhood provided the soil for a new, extraordinary development. Under the skillful guidance of Hitler and Goebbels, Nazi ideologists persuaded large segments of the depression-ridden citizenry of the Weimar Republic to embrace racial doctrines of spurious moral and scientific worth. The Nazi program was to build through blood and violence, if necessary pure Aryan "*Volk*," a warrior community led by an elite of blond supermen. In retrospect, Nazi beliefs are astoundingly incredulous, but at the time and in the grim climate of economic and social disintegration, they offered a hope—however farfetched and delusional—of supremacy.

It is the function of any ideology to organize the common perception around certain shared images in the pursuit of a policy for collective action. What was distinctive about Nazi ideology was that it prescribed the biological perfection of the people as the prerequisite for social transformation and national glory. That the "Aryan" race, as such, did not exist (it was no more than a fallacy thrown up by the still unscientific disciplines of philology and anthropology) was no real obstacle. Nor was the fact that the biological perfection of any race—eugenics—was and remains substantially beyond the capacities of science. For as an ideology, Nazism generated a new national enemy, one that could be used as a rallying cry—the inferior races. In *Mein Kampf*, Hitler's political testament, he writes, "Anyone who wants to cure this era, which is inwardly sick and rotten, must first of all summon up the courage to make clear the causes of this disease." The cause in question was the pollution of the pure Aryan race with the inferior, degenerate blood of Jews and Slavs and Gypsies. And what the inferior races did genetically was mirrored in what they did politically and culturally: They contaminated and polluted the body politic. The ultimate "cure" was nothing less than the extermination of European Jewry and other "inferior" races such as the Poles and Slavs. The imagery of this vision of a purified world was medical/biological. Nazism metamorphosed into what Lifton called a "biocracy."

By portraying the "inferior" races, and most especially the Jews, as a "disease" upon the nation, Nazi ideology succeeding in making them appear what they were in fact not—dangerous and implacable. No objective evidence could be adduced for these propositions, nor was there any possibility of confirming it in every-day reality. But the iconography of the Nazi propaganda machinery made it appear otherwise: the Jew was everywhere depicted as physically repugnant, as sexually ravenous and hideous, as obese or anesthetically thin and frail. The images were always extreme and the physical and moral baseness they suggested made the disease metaphor seem like a reality readily confirmed by perception. Indeed, so thoroughly did image substitute for reality that in the wake of *Kristalnacht*, it was the Jews themselves who were made to pay for the damage—the disease must pay for its own cure.

It was, of course, the classic case of pathological "enmification." A defenseless minority was turned into a public "enemy" as a means of providing a sense of vitality to a policy that was rationally and morally bankrupt, and as a means of utilizing and mobilizing a disorganized and disheartened populace. Dehumanizing this "enemy" went beyond the extreme of what Erikson[15] has termed "pseudo-speciation," for the Nazi ideology ultimately depicted the Jews as something even lower than an animal. In the process, the psychological needs of a highly disturbed leadership were assuaged as it projected onto others the evil within itself.

But it was most decidedly not for these reasons that war was waged with the Nazis; Nazi racism had no part to play in the American decision. On the one hand, though it was widely known what was happening to German Jews in the late 1930s, no efforts were made either to assist them or allow them to immigrate. On the other hand, neither Americans nor the British allies were the targets of that racism. With regard to us, as opposed to the Russians, Nazi propaganda had it that we were misguided and duped, rather than racially inferior. No; the reason we went to war was to check Nazi military expansionism. That our enemy was manifestly evil, and easily characterized as such, was a propaganda bonus, not a cause.

We are still paying for the luxury of having had such a genuinely evil enemy. World War II was as crude and as brutal as any war today, but the clarity of the issues and the effective characterizations, or caricatures, of the participants strengthened the way Americans felt about and defined themselves. In a word, we felt good about ourselves. Some of the moral and psychological premises that grew out of the war have continued to shape the attitudes of Americans toward their military involvements in the postwar world. Americans have come to see themselves as a new kind of warrior-hero whose best qualities emerge in wartime; the image, popularized in countless media products, embodies the following assumptions:

1. Behind every war in which America is involved is a moral impulse that justifies its participation—even if the causes are unclear or dubious.
2. Military combat has character-enhancing qualities. War teaches truths about oneself and others impossible to learn in any other way.
3. The very foreignness of enemies is proof of their inherent potential for evil. Only foreigners who have acquired American cultural values are tolerable.
4. American objectives in war are never selfish or chauvinistic. Americans are better, friendlier, and more accepting of others than anyone else.
5. In war, Americans are better fighters and have a stronger will to win than others.
6. As proof positive of their essential altruism, bravery, and willingness to prove themselves in the crucible of combat, Americans are willing to fight anywhere in the world where they are needed.

The books, films, and television programs that convey these messages typically make no pretense whatsoever at offering a political analysis of war. War is reduced to a personal drama in which the individual explores his relationship to himself, to his family, friends, and comrades, and ultimately, to a misty sense of patriotism. War minus its political and economic complexities becomes the individualized melodramas of Rambo, the Green Berets, and the hard-as-nails Clint Eastwood/John Wayne supersoldier. The iconography of war becomes focused around intensely lonely struggles, around tests of will and character; conspicuously absent from these standard scenarios is any examination of the institutional interests of competing political groups that derive benefits from war-making.

There is no question that this aspect of the American self-image—the all-American soldier—became solidified during the Second World War and has persisted as a dominant cultural motif ever since. That there is self-inflation involved is obvious. What is not so obvious, perhaps, is that this self-portrait cannot stand by itself. What is needed is an enemy. This the Russians were obliged to provide us with in the postwar world.

It should strike us how easily America's alliances shifted in the postwar period. Not only did West Germany become part of the Nato military consortium, and the recipient of Marshall Plan aid, but Nazi rocket scientists were greedily snapped up for the American missile program. Indeed, it now appears that even Nazi social scientists were enlisted by prestigious American universities for their think tanks. How, after a war of unprecedented destructiveness, did it prove so easy to ally with former enemies? On one level the answer is simple: Because there was a *new* enemy. On another level, we have to reckon with the delusory tenets of the American myth of the warrior-hero. Having defeated the enemy, Americans believed that the dangerousness had been taken out of him. The beliefs in American goodness and in American power led readily to the assumption that West Germany, at any rate, had somehow become a part of us. And so Soviet proposals for a unified *but unarmed and neutral* Germany fell on deaf ears. But the Soviets were now the enemy—and scarcely to be trusted.

Styles of "Enmification" in the Cold War

The shift from the Nazi menace to the Soviet threat took place with incredible rapidity. Scarcely was the Second World War over when our former ally, Uncle Joe Stalin himself, came to be cast in the role of a monster, worse perhaps then even Hitler. And again, any objective appraisal would have to conclude that Stalin was indeed a monster, one whose crimes have even yet to be fully cataloged. But Stalin himself did not become the "enemy" on record; that honor fell to something new in the American political imagination: international communism.

The political reality was that following the war, the United States and Russia emerged as clearly the two most powerful nations on earth. But the political regime inside the Soviet Union, though it pursued the same foreign policy objectives that it had previously obtained under the czars, was characterized by both methods and rhetoric that were quite unlike our own, and different again from that of the Nazis. Initially, it was not easy to get a handle on the significance of the differences. Marxist notions of the inevitability of class conflict sat side by side with Leninist principles concerning revolutionary political organization in an ideological mixture quite alien to American sensibilities. Even for the thoughtful American strategist, it was not easy to derive from official communist ideology either a clear picture of Soviet national aims and interests or a basis for engaging in a mutual dialogue. Moreover, quite unlike the Nazis, communist ideology was careful to advance the proposition that there is no such thing as an "enemy people." Lenin[16] himself wrote:

> The Socialists of the oppressed nations must particularly fight for and maintain complete, absolute unity (also organizational) between the workers of the oppressed nation. Without such unity, it will be impossible to maintain an independent proletarian policy and class solidarity with the proletariat of other countries in the face of all the subterfuge, treachery, and trickery of the bourgeoisie; for the bourgeoisie of the oppressed nations always converts the slogan of national liberation into a means for deceiving the workers. (p. 8)

There is a complex dynamic between press, government, and public. The government creates events and attempts, through propaganda, to impose interpretations of these events on the public.

The media do not create events for forefronting, but to some extent can select and interpret them. The government has more control of the *events*; the media have more control of their *interpretations*. But when the aims of government and media conflict, which has the greater influence on the public?

In the process of "enmification," the press is necessarily involved. But will it encourage "emnification" or will it restrain it? Again, we can see the complexities of the problem by seeing what happened in the Gulf War.

The Banks, Media, and Social Distress

> The Business of America is Business
> and whenever possible, Monkey
> Business.
>
> The reasonable man adapts himself to
> the world. The unreasonable man
> adapts the world to himself.
> Therefore, all progress depends upon
> the unreasonable man.
> GEORGE BERNARD SHAW

We live in a society that relentlessly attempts to litigate and legislate morality, yet the spirit of this age does not encourage morality. Such a situation inevitably results in superficial moral codes that dictate conflicting values. The attitudes of our times are the result of a social character that has, in a sense, overextended itself in such a way that everything has become possible and the rules of the game are constantly mutating. Morality is viewed as something we can invest in for our own personal profit, not that of society. This corresponds to Moynihan's idea of defining deviancy "down," which is related to our concept of social distress.[1]

Value confusion has become so much a part of the American scene that we scarcely notice it, even when it assumes ridiculous proportions. Consider, for example, the posture of today's banks. Not only is the depositor told that he has a friend at Chase Manhattan, but he is also regularly tantalized with the offer of free gifts. The bank ceases to present itself as what it was designed to be, a secure

institution that could both preserve assets safely and provide a
mechanism for investment.[2] Instead, it has become a kind of super-
mother, always there with supplies when you need them. In fact, the
banking community went so far in this direction some years ago that
there was a sudden alarming increase in the incidence of bank
robbery in New York City. The phenomenon is best described as
"bankrape." But the impact of this sort of offense pales beside the
wholesale plundering of the nation's thrift institutions by banking
executives. They, no less than the criminal with a handgun, have
abused the banking industry, considering it simply an ever-friendly
provider of gifts, a kind of Santa Claus or surrogate parent.

Lost in the banker-as-friend scenario has been any sense of the
dignity and responsibility of banks. In point of fact, banks are crucial to our economic system and we tamper with them at our peril.
Yet it is just this sense of the purpose and value of savings institutions that seems to have been lost, at least until it comes time to bail
them out.

No less important to the functioning of a modern society are the
news media. Here, too, we see value conflict leading to grotesque
distortions. News, having become a product, has to be made as
attractive as possible. The result is that reporters and anchorpersons
are selected for their attractiveness, while the real business of
informing the public is relegated to 90-second video-bites that do no
more for the viewer than provide a few striking images. Even local
news suffers as the studios learn that what the viewer wants is a
restored sense of community. Now the evening news is replacing the
hearth as a family gathering. It seems to manufacture news,[3] or it
attempts to do so, as the family once manufactured its own entertainment in the home.

What is really newsworthy necessarily has a social and political
context. But when the news media become producers of a popular
consumer item, they become functionally autonomous from the
society they should be reporting on, and the images they produce
come to drown out ordinary social and political discourse. The
possibilities for manipulation of the populace that result from this
have already been explored in depth in American national election
campaigns. But the problem is not confined to this country. Internationally, there is coming into being an entirely new form of mass-

produced culture—a "world culture," with its own distinctive features.

THE S&Ls

It seems difficult to pinpoint the origins of the confusion of values so prevalent in the modern United States. Just as the interpretation of descriptive terminology in the field of psychology has developed over the years, as we have seen with the case of psychopathy in Chapter 2, so have the interpretations of words such as "democracy" and "individualism" varied throughout the history of this nation. Peculiar to our modern times, however, is the confusion, ambivalence, or ambiguity of our codes of ethical behavior.

Consider, for instance, the traditional role of the bank in the community. The neoclassic designs of the buildings housing banking institutions provide the aesthetic elements leading customers to have faith in the noble keepers of their assets. Sober Doric columns steadfastly support the roofs of steadfast, reliable organizations. To challenge such an institution used to be unthinkable, except perhaps to the petty small-time bank robber. As a result of the coming together of these criminals, organized crime became the major force against the system. But the Mob of the days of Prohibition never operated from the inside of the institution, as organized criminals do today. The scandals surrounding over 400 savings and loans institutions in the United States today were for the most part "inside jobs." The Mob of the twenties and thirties was considered by the populace to be an organization that proceeded illegally and immorally. Mobsters could never aspire to being presidential advisers or Pentagon officials. This is not the case today, when criminal activity is found in the most respected and reputable positions in the banking industry as well as in the government.

The common man trusted the bank that would finance the kids' education, the family home, that very special vacation, and so forth. When a home mortgage was rejected, the bank's officials had a good reason to do so. This is no longer the case: A definite change in the image of the banks as conservative, highly structured, and carefully regulated institutions has come about since the early days of the

Reagan administration. The Doric columns now seem to be swaying to and fro in a haphazard rhythm while the last vestiges of trust and faith in the banks are blowing away. Again, we come back to the image of the sign that reads "No Trust" hanging in the barbershop that Melville created aboard the Mississippi riverboat Fidele.

In the early 1980s, the savings and loan industry was deregulated. Small S&L banks, thus allowed to deviate from their traditional role as standard mortgage lenders, began to create a more competitive market. These institutions took on a more ambitious approach by marketing an image of themselves as almost omnipotent. The bank down the street could do basically anything. For the customer, or rather the consumer, this brave new competitive market in the banking industry brought along fabulous benefits. Anybody with half a credit history could get a loan. And the banks went even further providing services, where the only regulation was coming from inside the system itself. The S&Ls were left alone to control themselves with their own conscience. It is not so truly surprising, then, that powerful bank officials, such as Charles M. Keating, Jr., of Lincoln Federal Savings and Loan Association, literally took the money and ran.[4] Nobody seemed to be checking up on what was happening inside the institution. So along with the benefits of the new and more flexible banking system, the customer has lately also been undergoing added stress because of the questionable reliability of the almighty banks.

Federally insured S&Ls are audited annually by independent accountants and are classed in four different categories according to the fairness of their financial statements: unqualified, qualified, adverse, and disclaimers. In the case of the Beverly Hills Savings and Loan, the appointed auditor was one of the most prominent accounting firms in the country, Touche Ross and Company. BHSL was taking excessive risks by funding speculative purchases of real estate that would later be resold for profit, thus extending its services far beyond the scope of a standard S&L to those of an investment institution. Touche Ross characterized BHSL as unqualified, seemingly overlooking the fact that this institution was participating in ventures beyond its designated range as an S&L institution. The auditors failed to give the warning to stop the deterioration of the institution in question. The accounting expert, Mark Stevens,[5] in his analysis of the BHSL case, explained the implications of the bank's auditor's actions: "When the auditor's signature is based on a questionable audit, faith in the system is threatened." Yet Stevens concluded that the accounting firms are not to be held responsible for these horrendous results, since the process of deterioration began at the management level.

What underscores the psychopathic tendencies of the system is the fact that the components of it that are supposed to be watching for trouble—in this case the accounting firms—are really only looking out for their own advancement.

BHSL's "behavior," if you will, is surprisingly in character with the type of behavior distinguishing the true psychopath, as we described earlier. As this institution overextended itself, it seemed to be seeking rather risky thrills and was consciously and premeditatedly putting itself into a dangerous situation by breaking standard rules. BHSL's accomplice, Touche Ross, willingly (it seems) went along with the exciting venture of breaking the routine by disregarding its responsibility as auditor to inform the public of the truth behind BHSL's financial statements. The reputation of Touche Ross as one of the most respected accounting firms in the nation provided the perfect smooth image that would at worst postpone, at best totally impede, the unmasking of the crime. The skillful bank officials evaded danger signals pointed out by their own administration. The alarms had been repeatedly sounded by BHSL's internal auditor in numerous reports. The system kept going, however, "accidentally" shredding files, rationalizing its own deterioration, and persisting in a sort of delusion that it had the power to break the rules. Running on an inebriating power kick, it dissociated itself from its own guilt.

The social distress catalyst that was launched by the encouraging platform of the Reagan administration, that policy of "open the door and look the other way," created the perfect scenario for the weaving of this malignant institutionalized web, which has had the cumulative effect of eventually forcing what we have termed the psychopathy of everyday life to unfurl and disseminate itself to even the most trustworthy institutions. When senators were asked to intervene in the case of Keating's Lincoln Federal Savings and Loan Association, they avoided taking immediate action. The result was great losses for the taxpayers as the situation got more and more out of hand. Keating's S&L association collapsed at a cost to taxpayers of $2.6 million, one of the most expensive bailouts in history. Some senators had stepped in to intervene with federal regulators on Keating's behalf. "The Keating Five," as these senators have been dubbed by the news media, had received contributions from Keating and his associates to be used in political campaigns. The seasoned Democrat from California, Senator Alan Cranston, was reported to have received over $900,000 in contributions from Keating. Cranston was brought before a senatorial ethics committee where it was concluded that his behavior was "improper and repugnant," that he had "engaged in an impermissible pattern of conduct [that] violated established norms of behavior in the Senate."

Cranston stood before the Senate and delivered a shocking speech blaming his misfortune not on himself but rather on the corrupt campaign finance system. Considering that granting favors for political supporters is more or less commonplace behavior for a senator, Cranston asked his colleagues:

> How many of you, after really thinking about it, could rise and declare you've never, ever helped, or agreed to help, a contributor close in time to the solicitation or receipt of a contribution?... There is only one way out: Get money out of politics.

Cranston's account of his actions can be described, to some extent, as an example of rationalization and dissociation. While accepting his guilt in the matter, he blamed his actions on another entity, the Senate itself. At the same time, he excused himself from responsibility by pointing to the malfunctioning of the system. While Cranston may not be a full-blown psychopath as such, the same cannot be said for most members of the House and the Senate, since they do not and will not bow their heads regretfully and admit to their guilt in the widespread con game of political campaigns. Proof of this denial of guilt on the part of the Congress is the absence of a floor vote for this case, which would have forced all Senate members to decide on whether they believed Cranston's behavior to be improper. "The Keating Five" scandal certainly does not represent a new type of behavior for Senate members. There is, however, an understood implication that, while this type of behavior is indeed "bad," it is not all that "bad." The worst part of it is really getting caught. The other four senators in this case were given a slap on the hand and were asked not to do it again. This case is not the first of this kind and definitely will not be the last.

THE BCCI

The scandal surrounding the Bank of Credit and Commerce International and its alleged ties with various banking institutions in the United States, including the First American Bankshares of Washington and the Independence Bank of Encino, California, constitutes another case study of the malignant effects of institutionalized psychopathy on more or less innocent individuals outside the system. BCCI was founded in England in the early 1970s as a clandestine money-moving bank. In July 1991, regulators in Britain, Luxembourg, and the Cayman Islands seized the BCCI and accused what had by then become a worldwide organization of widespread fraud. The BCCI had been accused of helping drug dealers launder their profits and of underwriting arms deals in the Middle East, in addition to secretly purchasing American banking institutions. Its modus operandi consisted of enlisting powerful government officials into its organization in order to maintain a respectable public appearance.

Just as the fall of the BCCI exposed the largest bank fraud in history, the U.S. case against the BCCI and five of its officers has been the biggest money-laundering conviction in American history. The five men were sentenced to jail and the bank was fined $14 million, the largest financial penalty ever imposed in a money-laundering case. The bank put together a $40 million legal effort to try to defend itself and its officers in the case. Some officials of the Justice Department were part of this legal effort.

In this modern era, advances in telecommunications make the world smaller and smaller every day, allowing businesses to flourish internationally. The BCCI, which operated in over 70 countries, achieved tremendous results while spreading the virus of social distress by means of its worldwide venture. While international businesses have the potential to bring the world together in peace, organizations like the BCCI provide a new means by which a malignant web of psychopathy can extend through everyday life. What is even more frightening is that it took so long for investigators from so many countries to actually put a stop to this operation. The CIA has been accused of ignoring many leads that could have led to an earlier halt of this con game. Again and again, one has to wonder whether the institutions set up to protect the public from such enterprises are only watching out for their own interests.

In 1985 the BCCI secretly purchased the Independence Bank through a frontman, the Saudi businessman Gaith R. Pharaon. Independence's ties with the now stigmatized BCCI have led to its frail financial condition. Taxpayers might once again be called upon to bail out a federally insured institution that might collapse because of nasty ties to a group of con artists. In the ongoing investigation hearings for this case, Pharaon has denied any wrongdoing on his part. Independence's possible failure could result as well in the collapse of the First American Bankshares in Washington, an institution also secretly owned by the BCCI. Deposits at First American fell by $540 million in the third quarter of 1995, a decrease that the chief operating officer, Paul G. Adams, attributes to "a media barrage in late July and early August."

We saw in an earlier chapter that creative mental dissociative processes, on the one hand, may lead to greater productivity and creativity when under conscious control. It has often been the case throughout history that breaking the rules can lead to a more creative, more interesting product. To put it simply, challenging the establishment—as a genius like Galileo did—has always brought advances. On the other hand, mental dissociative processes, when misdirected and not under conscious control, may lead to destructive ends. The genius of entrepreneurs in our modern era have, in several instances, flourished in situations where institutionalized psychopathy could easily grow. Financial wizards, expert bankers, and prodigious lawyers are the major players in this con game. Constantly challenging the established rules, they create a new game where the rule is that there is no rules.

Clark M. Clifford, a distinguished former defense secretary, informal advisor to Democratic presidents, and partner in the prominent law firm Clifford & Warnke, put himself in a rather perilous situation: He had to try to explain First American's ties to the scandal-plagued BCCI, for which he might to a certain extent be responsible. Clifford and his protege, Robert A. Altman, made a deal with the help of the BCCI to purchase stock in First American's holding company, whereby they made a profit of nearly $10 million in less than two years. As chairman and president of First American, respectively, Clifford and Altman from 1981 on repeatedly assured federal regulators that the BCCI had no hidden interest whatsoever in their institution. When it was finally disclosed that First American was secretly controlled by the BCCI, Clifford and Altman might have found themselves at the end of the alley. Their explanation, however, was that they were duped by the Pakistani founder of the BCCI, Aga Hassam Abedi.

Clifford and Altman voluntarily resigned their positions at First American. They offered their resignation only after a long struggle and protracted negotiations with other board members and powerful Washington officials. Clifford and Altman have been described as "men of honor," protecting the bank's reputation by leaving. But whether their resignations can be considered honorable to any degree is doubtful. Their course seems an action taken to save face, to maintain a respectable appearance before the world, after they had engaged in a risky deal with a clandestine organization. They are indeed honorable men, relying on their intelligence and prestige to maintain their powerful positions, keeping their real self separate from their public self, and going miles beyond the cheating-on-your-income-taxes syndrome.

Throughout its investigation, the Justice Department has been dogged with criticism from the news media and Congress. It has been said that the investigation is lapsing and lacks coordination. William P. Barr, the attorney general who has been put in charge of the investigation, denied these allegations, asserting that the department is making headway according to the standard procedures. In order to maintain that standard, the investigators must be allowed to proceed as is usual in such cases, slowly and with great care.

It is painfully clear that the banking institutions of the United States, those supposedly trustworthy organizations in their steadfast, classically structured buildings, have been slowly decaying, victims of the spreading of institutionalized psychopathy within the banking system. Meanwhile, the public merely stands by, observing, bemused by the involvement of men such as Clark M. Clifford and Senator Alan Cranston. This passivity is a symptom of the public's lack of any particular set of values, any clearly defined moral code. It is the very thing these con artists have picked up on and are using to their own advantage.

The Media

The clearly static and enduring structure of classical architecture, the inspiration and model for the buildings housing most government and banking institutions, developed into something quite different after the fall of the Roman Empire with the changing mores of medieval society. Clearly articulated facades decked with rows of white marble columns were no longer suitable, or perhaps slowly went out of fashion. The builders of great Gothic cathedrals had various new goals in mind; clarity and conciseness were not among them. Huge panels of colored glass filtered the light onto a myriad of shades and shapes. Great halls filled with images of saints and virgins and crucifixes perplexed the eyes of the beholders of the grandiose structure. The designers of this unreal world aimed at seducing the masses into believing in something beyond the harsh reality of everyday life. Promises of heaven—given that one followed the doctrine—rang out and mingled with the ambiguous light.

The medieval Church had mastered a powerful technique that would allow it to control the feelings, desires, and actions of all who entered the house of God. The cathedral was not simply a place for prayer. It was a place for political discourse (rallies for the Crusades), for entertainment (the reenacting of biblical scenes and morality plays performed both inside and outside the cathedral itself), and for family events (baptisms, first communions, weddings, confirmations, funerals). From the moment of one's birth to the moment of one's death, the cathedral played a key role in almost every aspect of one's life. In medieval towns, the highest and most prominent building was always the cathedral tower.

By the twentieth century, the cathedral had become overshadowed by skyscrapers reaching up much higher than the tallest belfry in the world. The World Trade Center's Twin Towers now hold the place of honor in the skyline of Manhattan that the cathedral would have held in earlier times. It is no wonder then that it has been a prime target for terrorists.[6] And on top of the World Trade

Center, a radio antenna broadcasts music, news, sports, weather and traffic updates for miles and miles around the tri-state area. Radio and television have taken on a role in some ways quite similar to that of the medieval Church, capturing the attention of the masses by means of fascinating images and sounds.

During the Middle Ages, the Church oscillated between being in harmony and serious conflict with the governments of particular regions in Europe. While the politicians—the kings and lords and governors of various lands—had governmental authority, the Church, through its appeals to the emotions of the populace, had more widespread influence over the people than any other institution. The Church was, in contrast to the regional or national governments, a worldwide institution, spreading its Catholic (universal) doctrine throughout the so-called civilized world. Its approach was quite theatrical, consisting of a wide spectrum of gimmicks to capture the attention and support of common individuals who would decidedly be more prone to following the word of the Lord than the orders of some money-hungry feudal lord. An authority that cannot really be seen but must be believed in is much more powerful than any head of state. Fear of the fires of hell kept the masses in check much more efficiently than the actual bonfires or prison cells of any government's armies.

Many centuries have passed and the institutions controlling the world have changed drastically. Yet while in the West feudalism is a thing of the past and the Roman Catholic Church has lost its hold over the politics of the Western world, there are similar entities—dressed in different costumes, acting through different means—that are basically performing the same roles. On the one hand, regional and national governments establish and disestablish peace and order in various communities. On the other hand, the media depicts this peace and order or lack thereof to communities throughout the world by means of satellite broadcasts. One important difference between our times and the Middle Ages is the disintegration of one particular set of values. The family, as the base and foundation of society, has always been highly regarded as the first and foremost place for the supremely important process of learning and assimilating values by the children, who will in time become the future leaders of society as upright, mature individuals. Traditionally, the family is regarded as a rather closely knit group where each individual fulfills a given role: that of the father, the mother, the daughter, the son, and so on. Families remain the building blocks of the communities that have always defined nations and now define the media audience as well.

Such nuclear families have existed and survived throughout the centuries. Now, as American society has become more diversified, more tolerant and accepting of alternative lifestyles, we are witnesses to the tacit but certain disintegration of the highly structured traditional family. Just as the traditional banking institutions modified their functions to almost absurd proportions, so has the American family mutated in organization to such an extent that the traditional structure is no longer the rule but rather the exception. There exist families with single parents, divorced parents, remarried parents; children brought up by gay couples, by groups living in communes; children born of artificially inseminated mothers, surrogate mothers, teenage mothers. The list goes on.

Some years ago, the National Broadcasting Company produced a three-hour documentary shown during prime time that portrayed alternative family settings in filmed interviews with various families.[7] These situations were then discussed by a panel of experts that consisted of psychologists, psychiatrists, and social workers, among them the well-known Israeli-American sociologist Amitai Etzioni. This panel was to comment on the status of the American family, on whether or not the institution was in serious danger of extinction. It was decided almost unanimously that American families were not in bad shape at all, that they were simply undergoing a process of change and reorganization. The only voice of disagreement came from Etzioni, who repeatedly cast dissenting votes expressing his concern over the decomposing set of traditional values that he believed was leading to the breakup of the family.

It almost seems as if this program had been designed to soothe and calm any anxieties Americans might have had about the circumstance that one of the most basic and important institutions, the fulcrum of society, was and still is in a state of decay. The program was underwritten by IBM and AT&T, two corporations that obviously have a great interest in staying on the public's good side, although in sponsoring such programs they are really manipulating the public by rewriting the rules, by promoting a new value system that basically states that there are no values, that any alternative lifestyle is acceptable.

AT&T is the link to one's relatives on the other coast or across the ocean. It is no wonder that AT&T had such high stakes in a program to pacify its most important customers. IBM manufactures the high-technology equipment that keeps the media ahead of the game, bringing the latest news and entertainment to everybody's living room. Through a collaborative effort, these three entities (AT&T, IBM, and NBC) provided a rationalization of the terrible effects of the dismembering of the American family on society, a denial of the existence of the institutionalized distress and psychopathy in one of the most important places—the home.

The media have slowly replaced the hearth as the focus of the family. It began when radios invaded living rooms and became the substitute storytellers. By providing image as well as sound, the television invasion went a step beyond that of radio. As is evident from the case of the NBC documentary described above, the danger posed by the media does not stem from their innovative use of new technology. Rather, the media act as channels of social distress through their inaccurate rendition of facts, their irresponsibility in reporting the news, and ultimately through their manipulative manufacturing of information that they tailor to their own interests. In 1990 the highly respected journalist Fred Friendly was featured in a PBS documentary, a retrospect of his career. "The essence of the problem," he asserted in one of the filmed interviews, "is that the media have institutionalized greed."

Not that the work of the media is always destructive: The networks have "enemies" that are also enemies of the society at large. A report aired December 2, 1991, on the Cable News Network examined the financial negligence of various agencies that provide food to the starving peoples of the world. This report dealt in particular with the scandal surrounding Ronald Ruskus and an important U.S. government development agency set up as part of the Marshall Plan after the war to aid needy countries. To date, more members of this government agency than of any other have been convicted for the fraudulent handling of funds: billions of dollars never reached the supposed recipients in Third World countries. This organization, funded by taxpayers' money, is yet another part

of the problem, rather than the solution to the problem of institutionalized psychopathy.[8]

The media also do society a great service in ridiculing those
great media frauds, the new generation of television evangelists.
These characters have learned from the mistake that Jim and Tammy
Bakker, made and have devised cleverer means for defeating both
the government and the media.[9] The faith healer W. E. Grant has a
yearly income of nearly $6 million. Larry Lea, whose prayers are
answered when his followers give him money to give to God, has a
comparable salary. By far, the fastest growing television minister is a
man called Robert Trilton. He produces a melodramatic variety
show to charm the viewers and sells holy water and oil by mail by
means of a very sophisticated system that operates demograph-
ically. The Trilton theme was "God and Prophet," but prophet
clearly came first. Trilton brings home a yearly $60 million. Such
individuals are obviously a great threat to the media. They are
getting rich very fast. The media's critical reaction to the television
evangelists has made the public aware of this con artistry and is thus
a measure against the spreading of social distress. This measure,
however, is still guided by the news media's need to protect their
self-interests by maintaining their position as leader in the market of
mass telecommunications. The news media have learned, like the
evangelists, how to get support from the public by giving it what it
wants to hear or what it is told it wants to hear.

THE GLOBALIZATION OF MEDIA
AND THE WORLD INFORMATION ORDER

While the news media tailor their products to consumer demand, they also have power to manipulate consumer demand
through propagandistic and subjective reporting. For many Americans, criticisms of the motives and strategies for the anti-Iraq coali-
tion in the 1991 Gulf War—as well as analyses of the Iraqi invasion—
were largely the doing of an antiestablishment press and electronic
media, whose patriotism was attenuated by the drive for ratings,
which translated into corporate profits. CNN, NBC, CBS, and ABC,
the major broadcast networks, have come to symbolize much more
than merely the Fourth Estate. They are perceived as an influential

political power in their own right, capable of significantly affecting the public perception and understanding of government policies. The public has lost its confidence in reporters who may succumb to the temptations of financial profit and disregard their responsibility as objective sources of information on what is really going on in the world. In the eyes of an increasingly hostile national audience of news consumers who no longer trust the media, the Gulf crisis became another example of media imperialism.

The war crystallized conflicts that otherwise simmered and lurked beneath the surface of events. Media–government interactions are one such problem. Since 1945, there has developed an international system for the production, distribution, and consumption of information. As with other aspects of world culture, the global structure of informational systems has been uneven, reflecting the division between the developed industrial societies of the First and Second worlds and the Third World countries.

The flow of news is dominated by a relatively small number of news agencies concentrated in the West. Prior to the technological sophistications of electronic communications, Associated Press (AP), United Press International (UPI), Reuters, and Agence France-Presse, were responsible for most of the organization and dissemination of news transmitted throughout the world, excluding the Soviet Union. Eventually TASS emerged as the equivalent of other news gatherers and served the USSR and its satellite states. It is American news firms, however, along with the BBC, that dominate the production and distribution of film and TV programs communicating international news.

MEDIA IMPERIALISM: THE WAR WITHIN THE WAR

The powerful position of the industrial countries in the production and diffusion of media amounts to what may be called media imperialism. A cultural empire has been established, and weaker states are especially vulnerable because they lack the resources and technical skills with which to maintain their own cultural independence. Virtual control of the world's news by the major Western media inevitably means the predominance of a First World outlook in the information conveyed throughout the world. Attention of the

Second and Third worlds focuses primarily on crises, disasters, or military confrontations.

Media sophistication and expansion in the West have also meant that internal conflict over access to, and interpretations of, information relevant to public policy is a major issue. Unlike the situation in the West, some Second and Third World governments try to exert rigorous internal controls over their own media, ensuring that the "official" way of seeing things and understanding things is maintained, while denouncing biases in media coverage from abroad.

Because of its relative freedom of access, the Western media operate in an information environment sharpened by political demands for making data a free or public resource, or, in other words, a public right like air and water. At the same time, the commercial utilization of information has become a central force in advanced societies, and the exploitation of that information a vital political concern.

Media portrayals of events in the public arena have important social repercussions, more so than in the past, because of the sophistication of information technology, which makes political questions accessible to mass-audience scrutiny. Consequently, media help to set social and political agendas. They select, organize, emphasize, define, and amplify a vast array of facts. They convey meanings and perspectives, offer alternative points of view to official positions on any number of issues, and legitimize, justify, or challenge the status quo. In short, media structure the pictures of the world that are available to us, and, in turn, these pictures may affect our beliefs and influence our modes of action. It is these complex and influential processes that arouse so much anxiety about the role of media in national and international affairs.

The major media outlets in the United States were heavily criticized in the Gulf War crisis. Poll data suggest that the public saw the media as too often at odds with the government, too committed to a particular ideological posture in their interpretation of events through the editorial process. Media were expected to assume a neutral position in their reportorial roles and to mute their own political preferences, identified by the public as a liberal slant on the news. The facts about political orientations among newscasters indicate just the opposite, however. The media are scarcely a liberal enclave; the majority of news broadcasters exhibit politically conservative tastes and tendencies and have transformed news into a showcase of right-wing virtues. Yet a significant body of popular opinion about the role of CNN in the Persian Gulf crisis, where it installed a journalist in Baghdad, saw CNN's operation as nothing less than apologetics for the enemy. In the emotional roller coaster atmosphere of the Gulf War, the refusal of some journalists to align themselves with the celebration of the Bush strategy brought them under fire.

In view of the public's general distrust of the media, why was there an apparent tidal wave of public suspicion about journalists who were simply cultivating their professional instincts of skepticism and who refused to shamelessly promote the administration's view of the crisis or to buckle under the news censorship imposed by the Pentagon? Moreover, why were critics of the government's policy charged with anti-Americanism? Perhaps the explanation is psychological: It was a collective therapeutic act in which the bearer of bad news was blamed.

Those who offered a different perspective and engaged their topic seemed to be in danger of being misread or misunderstood as agitators or propagandists. Though it is an article of faith that everyone is entitled to his point of view, somehow a humanizing involvement in the plight of Iraqis suffering under the crucifying bombardment of allied air forces was construed as untempered anti-American extremism. The popular assumption about the role of the media seems to be that empathetic commentary exceeds the bounds of journalistic responsibility. The news report is not expected to be a nexus point for the critical examination of policy. Should it become one, the journalist is not perceived as an analyst of policy but as a counterinsurgent, a literary guerilla subverting values and seeking to make plausible a parallel version of events radically different from those officially endorsed. The journalist is not to assume the role of sympathizer for the opponent.

When asked about the restrictions imposed on journalists during the Grenada war, the theatre commander replied that media types tended to get in the way and had to be kept out of the battle areas for the safety of the troops as well as themselves. He also noted that, in any case, journalists would very likely not know what they were seeing, had they access to combat zones. Modern warfare is a high-tech, complex mix of air, sea, and land forces that function in accordance with intricate tactical plans incomprehensible to the nonprofessional.

What the admiral's impeccable military logic misses or ignores is this: While the media may not speak the language of strategists, of "force ratios," "envelopments," "flanking maneuvers," and so on, that does not mean its accounts are intrinsically subversive of the military project. Indeed, it is entirely possible that they may, through their nontechnical narratives of the dream and calamities of suffering, lend support to the use of organized violence as a means of solving problems. Nevertheless, the media render the invaluable service of describing events in everyday language; the public is then better positioned to judge policies and policymakers, and to consider whether alternatives to violent solutions might not better serve its interests.

The professional military and politicians understand more clearly than anyone is willing to admit that public opinion in a mass society is formed and activated in media markets. The institutionalized means of free and informal discussion in face-to-face situations characteristic of our political folklore and exemplified by the Continental Congress and the *Federalist Papers*, where debate on public issues were freewheeling and radically democratic, are now fragmented and all but eliminated. In lieu of this is a centralization and consolidation of the opinion process. Controls and constrictions on the technology of opinion formation therefore enable the formation of opinion to be manipulated and authoritatively constructed.

It is clear from the controversy between the military and the media that the military did its homework and studied the press far more carefully than the media analyzed the military. Media controls from Desert Shield to Desert Storm are reminiscent of weaknesses deplored in other, nondemocratic states even by censors themselves.

POLICING THE PRESS: SOME CONUNDRUMS

The cessation of the fighting in Kuwait leaves several issues unresolved. When Desert Storm was launched, the military seized control of the news using various censoring methods. These included what is euphemistically called "pool reporting," and clearance of broadcasts pieces through the Joint Information Bureau under the authority of the Public Affairs Division of the Theatre Command. This meant that most reporters had, at best, only an indirect experience of the war. Few saw the combat operations firsthand, unlike many of their older colleagues in Vietnam, Korea, and World War II.

The war-coverage system installed by the military was worked out by the Pentagon and Department of Defense during the Grenada campaign of 1983, where reporters were simply barred from the zones. No doubt it was the impact of vivid images of bloodshed and horror in Vietnam that had secured the antiwar movement's legitimacy. Given the sophistication of the technical and institutional apparatuses of the media industries today, it is quite understandable that the military should have sought to circumscribe the activities of the press in the Persian Gulf. Understandable, but not acceptable. The information flow made possible by the tools of modern journalism could possibly have threatened the security of troops in the field or inadvertently disclosed the grim consequences of the systematic, organized violence a modern war machine is capable of producing. Pictures and tapes of such slaughter and mayhem just might have weakened the resolve of the American people in their support of a military solution in the Gulf.

The complexities confronting the press and the military can be reduced to two questions. Can journalists be trusted to provide news without endangering lives or national security? Though it is widely recognized that there is an abiding need to observe certain precautions in order to protect the lives of soldiers, is it legitimate to keep the American people from learning about the conflict that affects them and those they love?

Several prominent journalists and news organizations in the United States have launched lawsuits against the Department of Defense, arguing that the military control and structuring of news reporting in the Persian Gulf violated the First Amendment. The outcome of the litigation will profoundly influence news coverage of national issues hereafter. Yet the press faces a dilemma. If, on the one hand, it is perceived as lacking independence, its reputation as a source of objective, authoritative information on major issues can be permanently tainted and undermined. If, on the other hand, the media vigorously assert their role as a disinterested source of information whose posture toward government must be skeptical and critical, the perception of an adversarial relationship with government may still further diminish the respect of an incredulous American public, which already tends to see the media as politically suspect.

The president's repeated references to Munich in his briefings explaining why we went to war were intended to invest the crusade against Saddam's "Evil Empire" with the moral aura of World War II. The rationale for the Persian Gulf expedition seems to have drawn out the totemic symbols of a struggle where good versus evil was less the object of hortatory rhetoric and more clearly a conflict between the good guys and the bad guys. As Huxley and Orwell remind us, whether as empire, superpower partner, or civilizing mission, a government unconstrained and unchallenged by the press either degenerates into a conqueror or loses much of its moral force and savor as an axis of humane values.

The crisis in the Gulf produced a climate in which government and the media seemed to be treating the consequences of the Gulf War as if it were a monarchy. "The war is dead," they cry. "Long live the war." The war within the war between the media and government is into its next phase. The stakes are high. The objective is the ultimate control of public opinion and world culture. In the final analysis, the means of control of public opinion means the ability to mold the thoughts, feelings, and actions (i.e., minds) of the peoples of the world. The dangers of this kind of operation were announced to the public dramatically in two popular novels: Huxley's *Brave New World* and Orwell's *1984*. If we are going to recognize the dangers inherent in this process, we must bring to a halt the massive process of denial that is so prevalent in society today. A natural psychological process already exists within the structure of society that can help us recognize and understand the serious nature of this problem. I have chosen to call this the social dream, and by that I mean the society's perception, through the mass media, of the unresolved problems that it has been incapable of handling. It is to this that I turn next.

5

DREAMS MONEY CAN BUY

> You only live twice or so it seems,
> one life for yourself and one for your
> dreams. You drift through the years
> and life seems tame. So one dream
> appears and love is its name. And
> love is a stranger who becomes your
> own. Don't think of the danger or the
> stranger is gone. This dream is for
> you so pay the price. Make one
> dream come true, you only live twice.
> Theme song from the James Bond
> movie *You Only Live Twice*[1]

> We are such stuff As dreams are
> made on, and our little life Is rounded
> with a sleep.
> WILLIAM SHAKESPEARE, *The Tempest*, IV.i.

We have observed the institutionalization of distress as it reveals itself in several personal and social phenomena. These include the pathology of normalcy, the social breakdown of the mass society, the loss of personal reverence, the decline of the family and the neighborhood, the institutionalization of the value conflict, and the elaboration of the seven institutionalized stressors. Throughout the preceding chapters, we have examined the extent to which certain degrees of normalized psychopathy have become a part of everyday life, as evidenced, for instance, in the character of various national heroes, spanning the outlaw of the wild frontier and the gangster of the modern metropolis." From characters like P. T. Barnum to W. C. Fields, Ronald Reagan to Charles M. Keating, Jr., the social conditions fostering the attitude constitute the foundations of American pluralism. The readiness to cast aside the veneer of respectability, exemplified by Mark Twain's advice to the uncertain, "When in doubt, tell the truth," makes up an indispensable mark of the American national character.

The political tolerance of our confused century, coupled with the intense economic competition of the capitalist system, nourishes an attitude of loyalty to one's primary reference group, accompanied by a willingness to exploit outsiders to the limit of the law. As we have already asserted, the United States—particularly the urban areas—hardly resembles any type of melting pot. Rather, this country has become a salad bowl that allows homogeneous neighbors to exist with one another in an ethnic patchwork. This process results in the hyphenated American, whose loyalties have been divided by the overall society.

As I mentioned in an earlier chapter, the objective disturbances in a society's mode of functioning produce social stress, while the term "social distress" refers here to the inner value conflicts that arise in the wake of rapid social change. We cannot ignore the precipitous increase of social distress in existing institutions burdened with ineffective value systems that inevitably propagate contradictory doctrines. This "modus operandi" is self-defeating and it significantly adds to daily stress, for the individual as well as for the society as a whole.

By examining our conception of social dreams, we will have a clearer understanding of the psychopathy of everyday life as it takes place in our contemporary society. As we will see later in this chapter, social dreams give us not only a portrayal of society's afflictions but also the possible antidotes for treating the societal disorder caused by the institutionalization of social distress. To do this, we must first describe exactly what we mean when we refer to social dreams. Later we will need to justify the assertion that our society dreams and unravel the significance of such dreams. Let us begin, therefore, by exploring the nature of dreams themselves.

DREAM LANGUAGE

One of the most fascinating areas in the field of psychology is the study of dreams. Considering the many questions that still remain unanswered, dreaming is a normal human mental activity that apparently takes place during a phase in the sleep cycle called rapid eye movement (REM) sleep. The name comes from the restless sleep that characterizes this phase, in which the individual's eyes dart back and forth beneath the eyelids. Dreaming seems to have a definite biological function. Experimental subjects were deprived of REM sleep by being awakened every time they were about to enter that phase of the cycle. When they finally were allowed to sleep without interruption, they spent up to twice as much time as normal in REM sleep. Yet a controversial question of a more speculative nature still remains: whether dreaming also has a psychological function. Despite the obscurity of dreams, we are able, under certain circumstances and conditions, to determine what our dreams actually might mean. Therefore, one intuitively assumes that when individuals dream, they are not only fulfilling a biological function but are also relating information to themselves by means of the dreams.

In the interpersonal realm, individuals use *discursive* languages to communicate with one another to describe and organize their environment. All natural languages are discursive as are the languages of logic, mathematics, and computers. Such languages consist of a series of rules followed by the users to produce an infinite variety of statements, each to be understood on one or more levels, literally or implied. By contrast, in the private world individuals communicate with themselves by means of a different type of language, a *nondiscursive* language, which also has a given set of rules and a lexicon of sorts, used to compose an unlimited number of mental stories, or dreams.

In the discursive language of everyday life and logic, a word such as "chair" represents the symbol of a chair, that is, the abstract notion of a chair. Likewise, the Arabic numeral three ("3") represents abstractly the concept of the quantity three, for instance, three chairs, three days, three inalienable rights. As we logically try to understand the world we live in, we use and develop discursive languages for communicating with each other. Discursive languages use symbols that have moved far beyond that which they symbolize. The word "chair" neither looks nor sounds nor tastes like a chair, and the Arabic numeral three (in contrast to the Roman numeral three) does not resemble the quantity three. Nondiscursive languages, however, do not use symbols in such an abstract manner.

Rather, the symbols are directly connected to their real and tangible counterparts. It can be assumed that more primitive languages were nondiscursive. Metaphors and analogies are to a certain extent nondiscursive means of communication that remain part of interpersonal communication. But it is the language of myths, fairy tales, and dreams that is paradigmatically nondiscursive.

Natural languages require a certain period of time for acquisition. Children seem to learn to speak a foreign tongue at a quicker pace than adults, not because they possess some sort of innate knowledge of the target language, but rather because their learning processes are more flexible than those of an adult.[2] A person who has not acquired or who has little knowledge of a given discursive language will undoubtedly have a difficult time understanding any communication in this language. Such is not the case with nondiscursive languages, since the symbols involved are generally not totally estranged from their referents and one could easily guess at their meanings. Certain theorists have asserted that aspects of all natural languages are universal, yet the data supporting this point of view are to date insufficient. Natural languages in many ways are very culture specific. A good example is the very complex set of formal and informal second persons in a language such as Japanese as compared to the practically nonexistent set in a language such as English, where the pronoun "you" is used in formal and informal address, to refer to one or more persons.

The universal aspects of nondiscursive languages, in contrast to the those of discursive languages, constitute a strikingly plausible set, since the symbols involved in nondiscursive languages are manifestly associated with their referents. There is evidence that the language of myths is pancultural instead of culture specific. Consider, for instance, the notion of the sun as a male entity related to power and rationality, and that of the moon as a female entity with mystical and emotional qualities. Not all nondiscursive symbols, however, hold up across all cultures. A *universal* symbol, such as fire, is labeled as such because of the intrinsic relation between it and that which it represents. When symbols are understood with a more abstracted meaning, they become more culture specific. Such *conventional* symbols include flags, crosses, and corporate logos. In addition, there exists a group of symbols referred to as *accidental* symbols. These are of an idiosyncratic nature, since they coincidentally connect an exciting vibrant incident or circumstance to a given sign. An accidental symbol therefore becomes very personal, in contrast to a universal symbol, which stands deeply rooted in our bodily make up.[3] However, it should also be noted that the Egyptian hieroglyph is not simply a symbol or a sign of things but rather a more dynamic, complex symbolic system of its culture and dreams.

Individual dreams, quite like accidental symbols, have great importance and significance for the individual. They represent the individual's communication with his or her unconscious self, pointing out the problems and restlessness related to his or her conscious experience. Although Freud was by no means the first to wonder about their significance, Freudian theory constituted a landmark in the analysis and interpretation of dreams. Freud gave the study of dreams a more scientific framework, as he established a point of view that accounts for the importance of dreams in our understanding of human nature.[4]

From the theoretical point of view, the human mind has three constituent components: cognition, emotion, and conation. All three play a most important role in our understanding of human behavior. Dreams, as an essential part of the experience of the human being, must necessarily share these components. A society works much like an individual; it behaves affectively and cognitively according to its sensory experiences. Discursive communication within the society takes place through the representation of scientific knowledge by means of objective and analytical nonfictional literature and documentaries. But society also dreams, so to speak, through its artistic expression, and such dreams are of great importance. They represent intrasocietal nondiscursive communication.

The states of sleeping and waking are bipolar elements that the human organism needs in order to develop an ability to exist cognitively, affectively, and volitionally as well as to assimilate diverse sensory experiences. Between these two polar states—being asleep and being awake—oscillate nondiscursive and discursive dialects. Human knowledge is a continuum spreading between these two states, passing also through the state of daydreaming or daysleeping, an intermediate state of consciousness. Dreaming takes place at a given level of unconsciousness, and it is at this time that the individual is informed—by means of a nondiscursive language—of the nature of his or her problems in order that they may be understood and solved.

When a conflict arises for the individual, he or she attempts both to represent and to discharge it through a dream. But unless the significance of the dream is pondered in the waking state, the full import will be lost. On the social level the same thing occurs: Emerging value conflicts will be represented in works of popular entertainment, and the audience will discharge its emotional reaction to those conflicts without full awareness.

MYTHS AND DREAMS AND LANGUAGE

Human intuitive and subjective insight about the self and the concrete and tangible environment differs greatly from human objective and logical insight about the so-called truth. Myths and dreams expose ideas by means of images rather than through logical linguistic and inevitably more abstract discourse. They are similar to but more elaborate than poetic metaphors, which introduce ideas by means of descriptive phrases.[5] Ernst Cassirer, in his study of myth and human consciousness,[6] shows how images have functioned in the historical development of knowledge. A genuine symbol, according to Cassirer, is substantially phenomenological for the understanding of ideas. Formalized psychological laws governing this form lend symbols their important characteristics.

Dreams are symptoms of the individual's disturbances, just as ancient myths were images determined by the necessity or urgency of conflict. The act of dreaming functions as a kind of symbolic process, revealing not only the intellectual and emotional development, but also the imagination and state of physical and mental health of the individual. Dreams can often be quite serious experimental processes in the mind. The dreamer attempts to solve something by allowing his or her imagination to play freely. The commitment to action in the context of dreams does not have the same meaning as it does in the waking state. Communication in the dream must therefore be oriented to a number of other factors in the individual's life.

When searching for the underlying basis of a symbol, one inevitably arrives at a dynamic complex rather than a simple entity. The meaning of a symbol never depends on a single element. Rather, it is a part of a Gestalt pattern for which the interpreter must search. Lawrence Frank points out that "every language expresses a conceptual formulation of the world and how it is believed to operate. Thus the structure of a language, its grammar, syntax, vocabulary, use of verbs, etc. implies the basic assumptions of a culture about the world, how the events of it are related and how the speaker participates in it as a human being."[7]

Discursive languages possess culture-specific characteristics that lend the users a particular way of looking at and describing their surroundings and their inner emotions and desires. Scientists, when interpreting discursive analyses of the world, must be aware of this fact. On the one hand, we, as human beings, are necessarily so connected to and in unison with our culture that no matter how rebellious we may be, escaping this cultural connection is practically impossible. This phenomenon is most obvious in our use of discursive languages, through our culture-specific use of language by means of idiomatic expressions and the like. On the other hand, we, as individuals, have experiences of separateness and eventually come to resolve the paradox when we accomplish or take part in a criticism of ourselves and our cultures. Human nature attempts to transcend culture and actualize itself by self-examination and criticism, a dialectic process developed in the waking state by means of objective discursive introspection. In the sleeping state, this process transpires when we dream, that is, when we subjectively communicate with ourselves by means of nondiscursive images.[8]

SOCIAL DREAMS: A DEFINITION

Just as there is a certain degree of controversy about the interpretation of individual dreams, so is there a controversy about the interpretation of what we have chosen to refer to as the *social dreams* of our postmodern culture. As mentioned earlier, a society "dreams" through its artistic expression. Throughout this chapter, I will limit my focus to the traditional medium of literature (particularly the novel of the nineteenth century) and the modern medium of film, although we could easily apply our methodology to other artistic media such as the visual arts and music. The time has come for us to reinterpret the significance of social dreams in light of the social structure of our contemporary world culture, keeping in mind the concept of social distress. Social dreams function as a nondiscursive language in which the society communicates with itself, just as the individual's dreams are a nondiscursive language in which the individual communicates with himself or herself. Social dreams express both the nature of the social problems and their degree of seriousness. Our aim, in what follows, is to decode the language of the American social dream. As individual dreams operate in relation to the individual, social dreams have the function of informing the population of a given society or culture about its unresolved problems. At some point back in time, the curious Pandora opened her mysterious box and let out the vile creatures, spreading social distress to the most trustworthy institutions. The social dreams of our times have the mystifying quality of being able to communicate nondiscursively how their conflicts can be resolved.

I have attempted in earlier chapters to introduce and theoretically describe the concept of social distress, as well as to provide various examples of institutionalized psychopathy, the malignant web that has spread to all levels of the structure of society. I am about to take on a new perspective, that is, to analyze the close relationship between psychopathy and social distress in terms of several recent social dreams. My task is to decode or interpret the nondiscursive language used by the creators of these social dreams, i.e., the authors and filmmakers, so that we may gain some insight as to what action can be taken.

My use of the term "social dream" is innovative because it relates the interpretation of an individual's dream to a body just as complex as the society at large. Yet while my term is new, the essential idea of the "social dream" is not. The social dream may also be conceived of as a contemporary myth. The Greek sagas of Sophocles and Euripides were the contemporary myths, the social dreams, of the ancient Greeks. Beginning with Plato's *Republic*, the literature on utopias has always aimed at establishing an idealized society where the inhabitants live happily and peacefully without any type of social distress. Such "social dreams" culminated in the late nineteenth century with the establishment of several socialist utopias, particularly in the United States. A more recent work of great literary interest is B. F. Skinner's behaviorist utopia, *Walden Two*, where the "social dream" of a psychologist comes to life in a fictional ideal community. The term "American Dream" refers to the quasi-utopian image of the United States that was internalized as a belief in equality and opportunity: An individual may "pull himself up by his own bootstraps"; a newspaper boy can become the next president.

A political or ethical ideology is a daydream of sorts, a highly developed and conscious wishful feeling. What we are aiming to describe here parallels a possible conceptualization of society's "unconscious" and its functions. Our definition of social dreams is intrinsically related to what Jung called the collective unconscious of the society.[9]

SOCIAL DREAMS: SOME INTERPRETATIONS

The complex set of cues and signals that appear to the dreamer as an image reflects the dreamer's personality structure. For the average individual, the dream process, so detached from conscious sensory experience and communication patterns, makes inaccessible a full appreciation of the implications of the dream itself. The same applies to a culture as it dreams. It fails to get in touch easily with the meaning of its social dreams. In what follows I shall attempt to engage in a rather difficult process, to interpret the social dreams of our times in which the theme of social distress and institutionalized psychopathy is most obvious. I will primarily use the medium of literature and film. Fully cognizant of the abundance of social dreams depicting the problems related to social distress and their possible solutions, I must also restrict my discussion to include only a few examples.

Let us begin by turning our attention to the novel, which has been the major literary genre since the eighteenth century in most literate societies. This genre reached its most popular phase in the mid-nineteenth century, when the great novels of Dickens and Hardy were published in the daily papers chapter by chapter. The readers waited with bated breath for the continuation of the story, which would appear in the next issue of the periodical. Novels were read primarily for entertainment, much as films are viewed today. They portrayed the spectacular, adventurous, and romantic experiences of fictional characters living in the contemporary society. Yet the most important aspect of the nineteenth-century novel for our purposes is the fact that between the lines of descriptive prose lay an intricate account of the psychological development of the characters and of the society to which they belonged.

Friedrich Schiller believed that the function of the novel is to teach morality. "In the story of humanity," he wrote, "there is no chapter that teaches the heart and spirit more than the annals of aberrations."[10] He calls on the reader, already an expert on human emotions, to reflect on the extraordinary emotional circumstances of the protagonist in the story he is about to narrate. Schiller asks that an analogy to ordinary emotions be made and that the reader assimilate each experience read about into his or her own moral code.

I will attempt to make a similar analogy, consistent with my definition of social distress as developed in the preceding chapters. In this way my interpretations of contemporary social dreams may profit society by giving us insights and directions toward better understanding our belief systems. This in turn may help us resolve the psychosocial tensions in our culture.

The expression "confidence man," an Americanism that dates back to the mid-1800s, is used to describe the professional swindler "of respectable appearance and address," who induces his victim "to hand over money or other valuables as a token of 'confidence' in the sharper" (*Oxford English Dictionary*, p. 804). Such behavior has been described in previous chapters as being characteristic of the psychopath. In 1857 Herman Melville published a satirical allegory of the mores of his contemporary American society, *The Confidence Man: His Masquerade*. The story begins on April Fools' Day, as the devil boards a Mississippi steamboat, the Fidele, disguised as a seemingly harmless mute. The mute stands before a crowd and writes his motto on a slate for the people to see:

> Charity thinketh no evil.
> Charity suffereth long and is kind.
> Charity endureth all things.
> Charity believeth all things.
> Charity never faileth.

At the same time, the Fidele's barber hangs on his door a bold-faced sign reading "No Trust." The crowd reacts indifferently to the barber, but attentively and somewhat amusedly to the mute because of his uncommon behavior. The story is elaborated as the devil puts on a variety of disguises and proceeds to swindle money and quasi-philosophical conversation from other passengers by gaining their confidence.

A multitude of linking threads to the contemporary scene appear in conscious form throughout *The Confidence Man*. Our own world is repeatedly reflected in the world aboard the Fidele, the stage for a menagerie of characters: Quakers, businessmen, Indian haters, philanthropists, Swedenborgians, farmers, and buffalo hunters. The barber's sign announces the rules of social commerce that prevail: Trust and charity constitute the character of the weak, that is, of those who are most prone to falling into the devil's temptations. In this world of masquerade, the Bible is quoted everywhere and the characters pose as anything but what they really are. Melville paints a motley spectrum of archetypes of his day, a new breed of con men, not fictional but factual, not as prophetic passengers in a dream journey but as part of our own reality. Such innovative and unapologetic swindlers remind us of Oliver North and Charles M. Keating, Jr., of Clark M. Clifford and Robert J. Altman. They are not hardened criminals; they are instead symptomatic of the psychopathy of everyday life. *The Confidence Man* is one of the earliest social dreams relating this problem to our society, describing this defect spreading throughout the American national character.

Joseph Conrad, a Polish immigrant who settled in England shortly before the turn of the century, had traveled throughout the world at a time when colonialism was an intricate part of England's politics and economics. *Heart of Darkness* narrates the story of a steamship captain's journey up the Congo River to an ivory collection station headed by an agent known as Mr. Kurtz, a character embodying the creative and brilliant mind of a paradigmatically psychopathic individual.

The tale centers around the demonic Mr. Kurtz, who somehow has created a society where he has become king of the natives in a most primitive and uncivilized place somewhere in the heart of the African jungle. The storyline depicts the society Mr. Kurtz has devised—its king (Kurtz himself), its subjects, and its location—as one greatly vulnerable to and completely driven by a psychopathic force. The Prince of Darkness penetrated the deepest, darkest, most primeval site, the heart of the jungle, and has emerged as the omnipotent ruler of a greatly distressed society whose members venerate and cherish their psychopathic leader. Yet Mr. Kurtz, the essence of fascination and interest of those who seek the heart of darkness, is destroyed by the very thing that he set out to conquer.

The lure and popularity of this social dream can only be understood in terms of the attractive qualities of the dark side. The mystical, powerful Darth Vader of *Star Wars* represents another personification of the seductive powers of evil. Conrad, through the haunting story of Mr. Kurtz's rise and fall, sets forth the basic human problem in a given historical context, the period of British colonialism. The same plot with a similar theme was brought to the silver screen years later by the makers and producers of the film *Apocalypse Now*, situating the story in a different frame, the Vietnam War. Vietnam epitomized the disastrous effects of institutionalized greed, causing the greatest destruction of human life and environment since the Second World War.

When analyzing Conrad's message in *Heart of Darkness*, we are compelled to look into the social structures that we ourselves have built, ignorant of whether they be for better or for worse. Edward Said, professor of comparative literature at Columbia University, points to a parallel between Conrad's tale and the exploitation and failures of colonialism.[11] I agree with Said's interpretation of *Heart of Darkness* on one level. The so-called First World has placed the Third World in danger by exploiting its peoples and capitalizing on its natural resources. The First World, however, is at the same time destroying itself in different ways, perhaps by more subtle and unconscious means. Yet the gradual but certain deterioration of our Western culture manifests itself in multiple facets of our daily life; in the degeneration of our moral codes, the decline of the family unit as the nucleus of the society, and the inefficiency of our institutions. Such deterioration is evident in the rise in crime, poverty, and disease in our most modern cities. Finally, the problems posed by *Heart of Darkness* do not merely reflect the failures of international politics; they also implicate characteristic traits of human nature in general. The spirit of the evil Mr. Kurtz lives in the darkest crevice of the heart of Everyman. It is a universal spirit, a persistent plague in our distressed society. As T. S. Eliot wrote, it exists "here, in death's dream kingdom/The waking echo of confusing strife."[12] Although theatre is not a major medium for the social dreams of our times, the recent Broadway production of John Guare's play *Six Degrees of Separation* deserves to be mentioned in our discussion. Guare based his story on the life of David Hampton, a young black man who not long ago caused quite a bit of commotion in some circles in New York City. The real David Hampton, the perfect example of the psychopath, had the habit of conning his way into restaurants, night clubs, even the homes of the rich and famous by posing as friends of their children and taking money from them. In 1983, after coming to New York City, he spent two years in jail for burglary. He insisted that he never cheated his victims, since they were always perfectly willing to give money to him. When interviewed by *New York Magazine* and asked about his opinion of *Six Degrees of Separation*, he asserted that he ought to be acting in his play and that he should be receiving royalties for it, because, after all, that play is the story of his life. Hampton rides on the Zeitgeist of the psychopathy of everyday life in our own culture. He consciously picked on the wealthy and the powerful and perceived himself as beating them at their own game.

Six Degrees of Separation conveys the confused and ambivalent feelings of a New York jet-set couple invaded by the artistry and finesse of David Hampton, who introduces himself under the alias of David Poitier, the supposed son of the famous Sidney Poitier. He tells the couple that he got to know their children while studying at Yale; they are bedazzled by his cooking, mesmerized by his stories, and, most importantly, very excited about the prospect of acting in his supposed father's cinematic rendition of the musical *Cats*.

David Hampton played on what his victims were very successful in doing in the context of their socially approved worldview. The most shocking aspect of Hampton's attitudes and actions is the fact that he pretended to be like them. He understood clearly that the way to "beat the devil" was a process of seeking out those people who were, in his view, engaging in the psychopathy of everyday life as a successful and attractive lifestyle. In the film version of this social dream, Mr. Kideridge engages in an important conversation with his wife, who is pleading with him to help Paul (i.e., Hampton). Mr. Kideridge believes that his wife has been taken in by Paul and says the following to her. "I am not a bullshitter, and I don't try to bullshit bullshitters." In effect, Kideridge was saying that he was not a con man in his own image, and he does not wish to con a con man.

Ultimately, the film version was telling us that we are all separated by degrees (6 in particular) from being victimized by others as well as being able to victimize them. Hampton went too far, however; hence his defeat. He was too tempted by his victims' wealth and prosperity, which eventually led him to break the law and wind up behind bars.

The success of *Six Degrees of Separation* demonstrates the interest of the public in the character of the psychopath. Guare's case study is beautifully accurate; the protagonist embodies all of the salient traits distinguishing the true psychopath. Hampton dares to enter a society he cannot possibly belong to, seemingly because of the thrilling rewards involved. His intelligent discourse and carefully premeditated mannerisms convince the most experienced judges, his very victims. Every one of his actions is motivated by an irreverent pursuit of power that has no limits, no boundaries, and, most importantly, produces in Hampton absolutely no guilt. Yet the most striking aspect of the play does not lie in Hampton's psychopathic character but rather in the portrayal of the social distress in the subculture he invades—the New York City jet set. Realizing that it can do nothing to help Hampton, the well-to-do family could be said to be in a situation of social stress, the main objective disturbance of which is represented by Hampton. The family, however, whose lifestyle has evolved into one heavily burdened with inner value conflicts, suffers greatly from social distress. It can do nothing to help Hampton, not so much because of the nature of his problems as because of the family's very own nature. The society these people live in takes part in activities quite similar to Hampton's. It is driven by an unscrupulous and limitless pursuit of power, in which guilt and remorse cannot be shown, lest it disturb the public image.

Film has become in our century what the novel was to the public of the eighteenth and nineteenth centuries. In the modern United States, film is today the most popular medium for the masses, much more so than theatre or literature, seemingly because of the easy and passive access that viewers have to it, as well as because of the spectacular and thrilling effects made possible by the magic of film. To the typical member of our society, to go to the movies seems to be much more entertaining than to stay at home and read a book. Since the filmmakers of our times have in their hands the most powerful medium today for the transmitting of social dreams, it is of great importance for us to view films in an active manner, that is, to analyze and discuss their thematic content. In many cases, a film is based on a novel or a play. In other cases, films have sequels or are produced as a series (e.g., the *Superman* films or the *Star Trek* television series). I will refer to such instances as recurrent social dreams, which—like the recurrent dreams of an individual—come back periodically to haunt us with their warnings about our times.[13]

The recent film *Silence of the Lambs* began as a very successful novel written by the psychologist Thomas Harris. It seems to be the story of the incarcerated serial killer Hannibal the Cannibal, although it is not. It seems to be the story of the serial killer at large, alias Buffalo Bill, yet it is not that either. It seems to be the story of an FBI trainee; however, that is also not the case. It is really a story about the failure of the criminal justice system, masked by a cast of fascinating characters. It depicts our failure to beat the devil. Each individual part of the system fails to get the job done and evil wins in the end.

A young FBI trainee has been assigned to a dangerous mission by her supervisor, a forensic psychologist. She must interview Hannibal the Cannibal, a very dangerous man, in order to obtain information on how to capture another serial killer who is out on the loose, kidnapping women, skinning them, and making clothes out of their skins. She does not heed the warnings of the forensic psychologist not to become emotional with Hannibal the Cannibal. Because of her failing to do this, the dangerous lunatic seduces her into helping him.

Every character seems to be more concerned with gaining more power in the structural hierarchy of their workplace than with catching the killer. Because of this lack of cooperation, because of the inability of each member of the institutions involved to carefully and successfully complete his or her part of the mission, Hannibal the Cannibal has a chance to succeed. All he needs to do is to figure out how to coerce each one to fail. All errors, no matter how insignificant, work together in the end to allow him to escape. Even under the best of conditions it is impossible for our culture to beat this process of incompetency in the different parts of our society.

In the film *The Ruling Class*, Peter O'Toole undergoes a delusional transformation. Confined to an asylum believing that he is

Jesus Christ, O'Toole suddenly finds himself in important financial tangles with his family. A helpful psychiatrist tries a shock cure in an attempt to speed recovery so that O'Toole can pursue his economic destiny. The confrontation goes awry and O'Toole's "cure" comes with a secret new delusion, namely, that he is Jack the Ripper. This charming film (an audience favorite) puts forth an immediately accessible moral: To function effectively in today's world, it is better to imagine oneself a murderer than a saint.

The television series *Star Trek* and the various movies based on it also express a recurrent social dream. The dichotomy and rivalry between man and machine, humanity and artificial intelligence, and emotion and rationality are personified in the protagonists. *Star Trek* bases its morality lesson on the ideal that in order to survive one needs intellect and emotion to provoke the right and ethical actions. The rivalry between man and machine, personified by Kirk the fallible human and Spock the infallible Vulcan, goes back to earlier social dreams such as *Metropolis*[14] and *Frankenstein*. While the machine is trained to reason, the human has intuitive behavior based on emotions, which the machine lacks. The starship *Enterprise*, a futuristic law enforcement agency, embodies both extremes and aims toward finding a balance between emotion and reason. Its ethic is not to interfere but rather to help in other worlds, and the inability to find a balance between cognitive and emotional behavior represents the main danger for the society.

A powerful example of the psychopathy of everyday life can be found in an actual event of the 1950s, popularly known as the quiz show scandals. At that time, two prominent quiz shows, "21" and "The $64,000 Question," were in competition with one another. The scandal involved Herbert Stempel of Queens, New York, and Charles van Doren of the famed literary family as key figures. Both prime contestants were revealed as cheats in collusion with the media, who set it up. Over 200 people actually purged themselves before a grand jury. Van Doren also purged himself by giving a false testimony to a grand jury, an act for which he was later convicted.

Joe Stone, former Manhattan prosecutor for 25 years and a criminal court judge thereafter, broke the TV quiz show case by getting key figures to admit before a grand jury that the players had been given the answers to the questions in advance. Stone, who has written a number of books on other and related issues, thinks that lying is endemic in our society. Lying has, according to Stone, become a growth industry that pervades almost every aspect of American life.

Pioneer actor and director Robert Redford in the 1990s created a movie about the quiz show scandals taking some dramatic liberties with the facts of the case. The movie was a great success in spite of its controversy.

POPULAR SONG LYRICS

Lyrics to popular songs in and of themselves are interpretable as social dreams. As a symbolic representation of the spirit of the times, a song lyric may indeed reveal the essence of a problem plaguing a given society. During the twenties, thirties, and forties, the musical mood took on the form of romantic fantasy. Songs like Potter's "Pennies from Heaven" reflect the wistful feeling that better times must come soon, that life during the depression was way too hard, that a sort of miracle can bring us to a never-never land. In the fifties, times of financial prosperity, Elvis sang of love and rock 'n' roll. The politically turbulent sixties produced the ballads of Bob Dylan. And during the carefree seventies it was the Bee Gees and John Travolta who sang and danced the nights away.

The seventies was also the height of the Cold War, and popular music did not miss out on providing reflectional social dreams for the society to ponder. It is unusual to find a title song for a film that has in its lyrics all that is necessary to interpret the social dream conveyed in the film itself. The title track for the James Bond film *Thunderball*, a sort of "dream within a dream," is one uncommon example that I wish to examine more closely. The lyrics are as follows:

> He always runs while others walk.
> He acts while other men just talk.
> He looks at the world and wants it all,
> So he strikes like Thunderball.
>
> He knows the meaning of success.
> His needs are more, so he gives less.
> They call him the winner who takes all,
> And he strikes like Thunderball.

Any woman he wants, he'll get.
He'll break a heart without regret.
His days of asking are all gone.
His fight goes on and on and on.
But he thinks that the fight is worth it all,
So he strikes likes Thunderball.

The parallels between Agent 007 and the nuclear bomb become more than obvious simply from reading the lines above. Bond *is* the bomb. They are both licensed to kill. In the title song, Bond is said to always run "while others walk," and the Cold War was a relentlessly escalating process. An individual that is always ahead of the game has not only more power but also the possibility to escape and be saved in the end. Bond also "acts while other men just talk." Like Bond, the bomb takes action and does not participate in the tedious peace negotiations. "He looks at the world and wants it all," continues the song, perfectly describing the greed that prompts leaders to possess control of the world by means of nuclear armament, a power that could instantaneously destroy the world as we know it. Bond "knows the meaning of success," as he is the most successful hit man, very much like the bomb is the most successful deterrent to war. Bond's "needs are more," as are the needs of the arms race, "so he gives less," in the way that the funds for the arms race were always more important than funds for welfare or education programs. One of Bond's most alluring characteristics, as the song continues, is the fact that "any woman he wants, he'll get; he'll break a heart without regret." This lack of conscience, this dissociation of guilt, also applies to the arms race. Any woman, any nation, anything that is inferior will be eaten up, destroyed by this mindless contest for ultimate power. It is Bond, though, who has the ultimate power, as "his days of asking are all gone." The fight is said to be "worth it all, so the fight goes on and on and on," because the Cold War did have very enticing financial consequences.

The Bond films are also a recurring social dream, most prominent during the Cold War period. (Consider also the spoof on Bond by Peter Sellers as Inspector Clouseau in the Pink Panther films.) Although the days of the Cold War are over, the Bond films, based on Ian Fleming's best-selling novels, are still enjoyed by audiences everywhere. There is something in the character of Agent 007 that appeals to just about all members of the society. The Bond film saga depicts the struggles between three major groups. The Western allies (including Her Majesty's Secret Service and the CIA) are juxtaposed with the Soviet Union, starring the KGB. But the major world leaders in espionage learn to cooperate with each other in order to save the world from a greater evil, the archvillain who leads an organized crime group (SPECTRE) that is prepared to take over or destroy life on the planet. These fantastic characters, who usually live in beautiful mansions and cruise around the Mediterranean in their grandiose yachts surrounded by beautiful people, are the real psychopaths (as opposed to Bond, who is the sublime and socially praised psychopath): they believe that their money will bring them power and control, that they will get away with everything. In the end, however, the forces of good defeat those of evil. The two opposing world powers unite to save the planet from a crazed lunatic with a warped ideology.

But if one follows the progress of the Bond stories over time, one readily detects a curious evolution in the figure of the enemy depicted therein. Whereas in the initial novels the enemy was clearly identified as the Soviet Union and its protégés, in the later novels the enemy has shifted in a seemingly fantastic direction. In *Thunderball*, for example, the enemy is an international terrorist syndicate, with access to all the fruits of modern industrial technology, intent on asserting its own hegemony over both the superpowers. Indeed, this syndicate, ultimately controlled by a single madman, has managed to dupe both Russian and American military planners. To defeat this enemy, moreover, Bond is forced to make common cause with a Russian agent. Nor does the progression stop there. In yet a later novel still, Bond passes from being the coldly calculating philanderer to actually falling in love with a Russian agent, no less.

It would seem that Fleming, in an intuitive and imaginative leap that is the artist's prerogative, has anticipated the age of Glasnost. But if this is so, we should note that his vision continued to make use of even more sinister figures for Bond to confront. And if we pause to consider what his imagined SPECTRE may represent, there is no reason for us to be overly optimistic about peace and "de-enmification." For in the criminal syndicate of the later Bond novels, we seem to have a personification of a curious fusion of international capitalism, mass media, organized crime, and renegade elements within the major military establishments. In a certain sense, of course, the portrait could well be of our own institutions. But in the shadow logic that pertains to the process of enmification, the threat posed to our welfare by our own institutions as they are presently constituted has been projected outward. It will be interesting, to say the least, to see how Fleming's scenario is played out in real life, to see, in other words, who the next enemies are.

This "war triangle," the main ingredient for any good Bond film, separates the three powerful entities by very thin boundaries. The role of the organized criminal cartel will greatly influence world stability. The transformations that this group will take are of the utmost importance for the future, as I pointed out earlier in Chapter 4 in my discussion about enemies. In a world where national character has become blurred by the development of an overarching world culture, ethnic rivalry emerges with the consequential international criminal organizations. This seems to be the status of the new world order.[15] The great political international organizations shrink in the shadow of their most destructive enemies, the drug lords of Latin America, the front men of the Bank of Credit and Commerce International, and so on.

Rollerball, a film very reminiscent, both in theme and content, of the two futuristic literary masterpieces *1984* and *Brave New World*, portrays an alternative world order set in the year 2018, where one world culture and six corporations, each based in a major city, have total control of the planet's population and resources. The people live in utter tranquility. War no longer exists, neither does violence or crime, poverty, or antiestablishment unrest. To allow the populace to let out its aggressions, a game called rollerball, an ingenious cross between roller derby, motorcycle racing, and basketball, has been devised. Players zoom around a sloping track on rollerskates or motorcycles and try to insert a heavy iron ball into the goal. The intensity of the action around the track involves violent aggression between the two teams, which often culminates in the bloody death of the players.

Jonathan E. has become the star player for the Houston team, which has remained undefeated in the last series of games. The Energy Corporation, which owns the team, appoints Bartholomew, one of it top executives, to order Jonathan to retire. He refuses to do so and embarks on a quest to understand why he has been asked to retire. This leads him to finding out that all the books—all the knowledge in the world—have been condensed into one gigantic database in the Geneva computer. Traveling to Geneva he finds the computer guarded by a frenzied fumbling scientist. When Jonathan asks the computer about the corporations, the mass depository of knowledge gives a nonsensical answer. All vestiges of individuality and desire for autonomy and knowledge of the past have been destroyed. *Rollerball* thus expounds a theme of human survival against mechanical as well as human machines, computers, and corporations. Jonathan's quest for understanding is, in a way, also a quest for survival. Knowledge seems to be the only way out, but in his society where the masses are so easily controlled by the media and television screens have taken over the minds of all, knowledge is but a thing of the past, forgotten by everyone.

The film climaxes with a game between Houston and Tokyo. The rules have changed, loosening the restrictions on violence. This inevitably leads to a massacre on the track, of which Jonathan is the only survivor. The victory goes to Houston. The mob cheers as it probably would have had Jonathan also been killed in the game. His efforts to understand and supersede the system seem to have no more of an effect on his society than the apathy or lack of insight of those around him. The main theme exposes the dehumanization and the mind control that may occur in a futuristic society. The moral of the story seems to be that society will stop any possibility of world destruction by means of the violent rollerball games; that is in fact what the game was devised for. The world order is quite simple: one world culture and no national boundaries. When Jonathan gets notice that he must quit the game and he says he wants to win in order to play the game as it should be played, Bartholomew takes him aside and explains that all of this has been done to prevent war. If Jonathan continues playing, the intricate plan devised after the end of the mysterious "Corporate Wars" will be undone. It is understood in this society that dehumanization is a sacrifice that one must make for the sake of world peace. *Rollerball* points out that our society is definitely going in that direction. For the sake of peace, our governments build up their nuclear arsenals. For the sake of peace, wars are waged on foreign soil. For the sake of peace, our Western culture has developed an intricate and extensive moral code stagnated with contradictory and inconsistent methods.

The imminent danger of artificial intelligence is another theme in *Rollerball*, exemplified by the scene with the Geneva computer. Both the computer and its curator have gone mad. Jonathan's quest for knowledge has been thwarted by an international effort to condense all information in a single source. The question of human survival when confronted by machines is an issue raised by this film that should and must engender concern among viewers. This theme is taken up in a different way in a recent TV miniseries entitled *Wild Palms*, created by Oliver Stone.[16]

In the early 1970s, a film, *The Stepford Wives*, and its sequel, *The Return of the Stepford Wives*, portrayed in a futuristic setting the battle of the sexes. In a small Westchester town, whose inhabitants are seemingly normal young professionals leading normal lives, joining country clubs and acquiring various goods, a mysterious plot against women is taking place. The men have decided to take revenge on their liberated wives and have worked out a strategy to totally change them into obedient, subservient housewives. A young couple moves to the town, unaware of the situation. The men's group enlists the husband but the wife resists, becomes suspicious, and goes for help. In the sequel, it is the women that take revenge by a more violent method: by killing the men.

These two films exemplify not so much the inequalities between the sexes as the actual struggle and disagreement that is still going on. This social dream then warns of disintegration of the family as well as of the blurring of male and female roles, which are crucial for the survival of the family. There is an unannounced war between women and men, and we cannot disregard the urgent need for a sane solution. The struggle must be worked out before the two sexes unwittingly undermine the very foundation they each need, that is, the love and cooperation between women and men, a most necessary ingredient for the survival of the family.[17]

COMMERCIALS, COMICS, AND FILM CARTOONS

During the 1960s and 1970s, a public service commercial funded by the College Boards and Educational Testing Service was aired. Devised by a Madison Avenue advertising firm employing quite exemplary social dreamers, a short commercial was produced in two different versions. It aimed to convince individuals with life experience to go back and obtain high school diplomas. Open enrollment was then a new program for educational institutions. The mores of the educational system were changing. The first version of the commercial was set in a dingy office, where a man sat at his desk eating a corned beef sandwich. Enter Abe Lincoln, dressed in top hat, black suit, etc.

> MAN. Name?
> ABE. Abraham Lincoln.
> MAN. Have a seat. (*Abe sits.*) Got a driver's license?
> ABE. No ... I can't drive ...
> MAN. High school diploma?
> ABE. Uh ... I educated myself ...
> MAN. Abe, you ain't gonna get nowhere without credentials, y'know what I mean?
> (*Exit Abe. End of commercial.*)

This interesting but puzzling ad did not get good results from the viewers, since the message was somehow hitting the wrong target. Instead of convincing people to enroll in education programs, it was pointing a finger at the collapsing educational system in the United States. If Abraham Lincoln cannot make it without a degree, what is the individual with normal intelligence and motivation to do? Recognizing their mistake, those involved with this promotion devised a second version of the commercial that aired for quite a long time. This new version is set in a classroom where a teacher discusses the Civil War with his students. Abe Lincoln walks in and sits down. The message is already clearer and more positive, as Lincoln has decided to go back to school. As the teacher asks questions, Lincoln immediately raises his hand and answers correctly every time. The teacher, either ignorant of Lincoln's identity or indifferent to it, says, "Very good, very good," and the commercial ends. Lincoln is never identified by name in either version of the commercial.

These ads are, unwittingly it would seem, revealing some of the greatest problems with the educational system of the United States. We are unwilling to recognize people for who they are. We seem merely to want paperwork. It is more important in this society to have the correct credentials and a laser-printed CV (with impressive facts about one's life) than to actually have the motivation and the experience that the impressive resume is supposed to represent. If something on paper is wrong, inadequate, or missing, the individual will no longer be considered—not even looked at. When individuals are no longer recognized for who they are, the society is moving into one more phase of the processes leading to dehumanization and alienation. The abstraction of an individual by means of test scores and the like has become overhauled, more important than the real individual and his or her real abilities.

The amazing Superman provided subject matter for a comic book, a film, a television series, and later on another film with two sequels. In the golden age of comics, Superman became the most popular superhero, a sort of "archsuperhero" defeated by none, respected by all. This epic character emerged in 1938, just as the United States was on the verge of entering the Second World War. But the quest for a *"ganz amerikanischer Ubermensch"* comes out of an earlier period, the turn of the century, after Nietzsche had introduced his philosophical ideal.

Nietzsche's term *Ubermensch*, literally translated as "above-human," referred to a person with the rational and emotional capacity and the volitional need to transcend the problems of Nietzsche's society, somebody above (*uber*) all of the societal nonsense. The Americanized version of the *Ubermensch* mutated into a different concept. In George Bernard Shaw's *Man and Superman*, Dona Ana, Don Juan's mistress, utters the illuminating last words of the play:

> ANA. Where can I find the Superman?
> DEVIL. He is not yet created, Senora.
> ANA. Then my work is not yet done … a father—a father for the Superman.

She aims not to become a superman herself. Rather, she has developed a passive attitude that hopes for the coming of a particular type of savior, the superman, a creature better and more trustworthy than any ordinary man.[18]

In the American society of the late 1930s, so concerned about the Depression and the emerging problems in Europe, there materialized a strong feeling of necessity for a superman. A far cry from the Nietzschean ideal, the American superman represented the benevolent, all-powerful figure who would deliver the American people from the evil in the world, like the good king in fairy tales who would always help his subjects and distribute wealth fairly. In a land where kings are unconstitutional, the people of the United States looked to outer space and found their idol in Superman, the alien from the planet Krypton, who came to a world about to hit rock bottom and had the power to save it.

The comic strip, a very dynamic form of communication, qualifies as an ideal medium for social dreams. Growing out of the humorous cartoons of the late nineteenth century, (some political, others simply social satires) the "funnies" are as American as apple pie. "The Katzenjammer Kids" was the first American comic strip, introduced by Rudolph Dirks, a German immigrant, in 1897. Dirks went to New York City in search of a job as a cartoonist, and Rudolph Gluck, the comic strip editor for the Hearst-owned newspaper the *New York Journal*, hired him to do something based on the illustrated children's storybook *Max und Moritz*, published in Germany in 1855. "The Katzenjammer Kids" contributed to the growth of the Sunday paper in American journalism. They proved to be a sensational success, rising to an all-time high at the turn of the century. Hans and Fritz, the two little hangover[19] devils, took America by storm.

The great entrepreneurs Joseph Pulitzer and William Randolph Hearst invested heavily in the new medium of the comic strip and set up a very competitive arena. The comic strip became a colorful weapon in the paper circulation wars of late nineteenth- and early twentieth-century journalism. The comics were not only for children; they also appealed to adults and, most important, to American adults living in a very ethnically diverse society. Thus comic strips have as their major target the hyphenated American. The bait-readership, the bid for higher circulation devised by the owners of these papers, was to appeal to millions of immigrants who were arriving by ship each week from all the corners of the world.

The immediate success of "The Katzenjammer Kids" greatly increased the readership of the *New York Journal*. Dirks and Gluck, however, had constant battles caused by their clashing personalities. These feuds culminated in Dirks's acceptance of an offer by the Pulitzer-owned *New York World* in 1912, a defection that resulted in a lawsuit that made front-page news all over the country. The legal proceedings, including several appeals, continued up to 1919. In the interim there were variations on the theme of "The Katzenjammer

Kids," of course, under different names because of the trademark suit. Dirks continued a strip called "The Captain and the Kids" for the *World*, while the Hearst paper hired H. A. Knerr to draw a strip under the name of "Hans and Fritz" until the lawsuit was settled. After the lawsuit, the *Journal* was awarded the name "Katzenjammer Kids" drawn by Knerr and the *World* continued its "Captain and the Kids" drawn by Dirks.

The stories of the two little hangover devils had a worldwide appeal, evidenced by their longevity, as their popularity lasted up until 1980. Dirks died in 1949 and Knerr in the late 1960s, but the strip was continued by other artists. Their powerful message was disseminated not only by the Sunday funnies, but also as the subject matter of several separately published books, as the theme of buttons found in cereal boxes for kids, as the topic of various games and puzzles, and finally as the motivation of silent and eventually sound cartoons. Versions of the "Katzenjammer Kids" quickly became popular in Scandinavia, Italy, England, and even Israel.

The stories about the adventures of these two nasty little boys announced the danger of what may happen in a society where the family has collapsed and a counterdependent attitude toward authority is present. The two kids, Hans and Fritz, engage in antisocial behavior, playing pranks on the authoritarian male figure. They live with their mother and the Captain, an old sea dog who came to live with the family in 1902. Poppa Katzenjammer, who played a minor, passive role during the first few years of the strip, quickly disappeared, and Momma was left as the first popular single parent in an American cultural medium. The public seemed not to recognize the significance of the corruption inherent in this one American family, where the boys steal Momma's pies and put firecrackers under chairs. The Inspector, an old friend of the kids' father, steps in as another authority figure, also disrespected by the kids. The main characters speak in a pidgin German dialect and a cast of supporting characters represents the multiple ethnic groups who immigrated to the United States during the era the comic strip was at its height: the Chinese cook and some of the Captain's sea mates, the Italian and Irish neighbors, and so forth.

The psychological dynamics depicted by the characters of Hans and Fritz exemplify the popular notion that "boys will be boys," also reminiscent of the "Peck's Bad Boy" character, the subject of many early silent films. There is in the kids' personality a counterdependent and irrational resentment of authority. Hans and Fritz represent the psychopathic character in development. They fulfill the three characteristics of the psychopath (see Figure 5.1). Their outward appearance is not mean, as Momma always calls them her "little angels," although this is indeed a false representation of them, passing on as something they are definitely not. They participate in violent antisocial behavior, which for the reader is quite humorous, although it has inherently distressful social implications. The kids, in a way similar to that of the psychopath, seem to be thrilled in the face of danger and seem not to fear the consequences, usually a terrible spanking by the Captain.

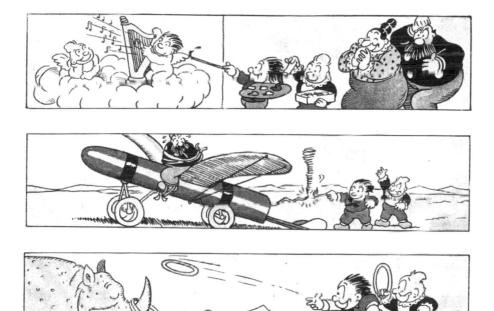

FIGURE 5.1. (top) The sincerely insincere kids falsely present themselves as angels when in reality they are perfect devils. (center) Totally capable of blowing away the captain, the kids manifest their dangerous, violent lifestyle. (bottom) Practicing their thrill-seeking needs, the kids illustrate their irresistible fascination with the game of danger. The kids rush in where angels fear to tread. (Reprinted with special permission of King Features Syndicate.)

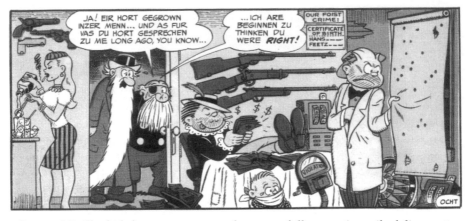

MAD Magazine did a spoof on the Katzenjammer Kids (see Figure 5.2), giving the reason why its popularity died out. They asserted that the kids had never grown up in the strip.

MAD created a new strip, where Hans and Fritz, in their teens, have become juvenile delinquents. The kids have taken over, and the family, as the nucleus of society, has lost all power to deter the kids' antisocial behavior.

Basing itself on the children's book *The Fifty-First Dragon*, U.P.A. created a very humorous cartoon portraying yet another very meaningful social dream. U.P.A., the alternative to Walt Disney cartoons, rendered to the public the tragicomic story of Glenn, the boy who decides to go to "knight school" because he wants to be a great hero. Glenn's attitude fits in with the tradition of the superman or superhero, stemming back to the Wagnerian myths of the latter part of the nineteenth century. He takes Dragon-Killing 101, where he realizes that he is rather afraid of dragons, that he is more of a coward than he thought. His wise professor, however, gives him some good advice and encourages him to go on with his endeavors. He also gives the cowardly Glenn some extra protection. The professor tells him a magic word, "rumplesnitz," which, when uttered in the sight of a dragon, will supposedly shield the speaker of the word from any harm done to him by the dragon.

And so Glenn goes off to fight some dragons. He kills many and becomes quite famous, greatly adding prestige to the knight school where he was trained because of his wonderful accomplishments. Glenn, however, has a tragic flaw. He likes to celebrate and drink pints of ale with his buddies, especially when returning home from his dragon-killing excursions. When he has killed his fiftieth dragon, he goes to the tavern and spends the night drinking and dancing, disregarding the fact that the next day he must face a most terrible foe, the fifty-first dragon.

The next morning, his friends have to pull Glenn out of bed and lead him to the cavern where the dreaded dragon waits. Glenn is half asleep and still quite drunk when he encounters the dragon. Glenn takes out his sword and gets in the fighting position only to realize that he has forgotten the magic word! He stands there, speechless, not knowing what to do, overcome by a great fear, and the dragon asks him, puzzled, "Say, knight, what's a matter with you?" By reflex, Glenn flings his sword at the dragon and kills him instantly. He panics, though, when he realizes that he has not said the magic word.

A very depressed Glenn, now no longer partaking in knightly acts, runs into his dragon-killing professor. He accuses the wise old man of being a cheat, asserting that the magic word gimmick was a hoax, declaring that the man lied to him. Glenn has disgraced the school by proving himself to be a no-good dragon killer. His days of fame and glory are over, and so he goes to bed and refuses to get up anymore. His friends and colleagues force him out, hoping he will return to his dragon-killing, which had until then been the best in the county. But when he gets up, he leaves town and is never heard from again.

A major flaw in the American national character stands parallel to Glenn's self-destructive attitudes and resignation in the face of danger. That feeling of hope for the superman magic, the motivation to do something without taking full responsibility for one's actions, causes great failures in the system. The vast majority of the public will believe more in something seen on television than in something seen with its own eyes. People are afraid to live life, and get vicarious pleasure from watching the soaps. Americans seem to be looking for the hero who will save them, and they are ready to pay any amount of money for the gimmick, the product, the shortcut to make it without a full-hearted effort. The social dreams of our times seem to be screaming out, proclaiming this problem to us, yet nobody seems to be listening. The public lacks the sense of responsibility to listen to the lessons that even the most popular media are begging it to recognize.

At this point it would be worthwhile to analyze the media's role in disseminating information regarding the problem of crime and justice in the courtroom. Americans seem to have developed an obsession with the symbolic value of being a victim. Playing the victim can hide a perpetrator from the consequences of both normalized psychopathy and more serious criminal acts, even murder. In 1994, Alan Dershowitz coined the term "abuse excuse" to describe the legal tactic by which criminal defendants claim a history of abuse that exonerates them from violent crime. In Dershowitz's argument, largely inspired by the Menendez brothers' murder trials (both used sexual molestation by the victim as their defense), the "abuse excuse" reached its peak as a license to kill. Another example of the "abuse excuse" may be found in William Kunstler's hypothetical but unused "black rage defense" for Colin Ferguson, the man who killed and maimed commuters on the Long Island railroad shortly before Christmas in 1993.

There are many other examples that continue to be covered by the media. Law suits of all types seem to be coming out of the woodwork, for example, false memory syndrome litigation and U.F.O. survival syndrome. With an atmosphere of circus mania, litigations seem to be the Zeitgeist of our time. In the Menendez case, for example, the defense put the victims (Kitty and Jose Meendez) on trial. Jose was the evil controlling father and Kitty his docile coconspirator. The defense wanted jurors to believe that Kitty and Jose drove their sons to murder and that they therefore should not be responsible for their actions. The Bobbitt case, which took place in the context of an already existing war between the sexes, provided a fine example to illustrate the growing tendency of normalized psychopathy and social distress within our society.

Lorena Bobbitt, who severed her husbands penis while he was sleeping, was portrayed by many women as a folk hero. Most of the information seems to confirm that John Bobbitt, Lorena's husband, did not threaten to hurt her if she left him. Furthermore, there was ample evidence that he actually wanted to leave her. Lorena had a fairly good income and no children at the time of the incident. There was a general tendency among women within as well as outside the feminist movement to legitimize her crime. John Wayne Bobbitt also emerged as a victimized folk hero through vulgarized media promotions when he appeared in a XXX pornographic movie titled "John Wayne Bobbitt Uncut."

The above facts have stimulated me to develop a research project that investigates the effects of both Bobbitt case decisions on the attitudes of college students with regard to their future interpersonal sexual relationships. My hypothesis was that groups of students expressing their feelings about the Bobbitt case decisions would differ significantly while in conversation with one another. In order to test this hypothesis, I set up three groups who were instructed to engage in conversations regarding their attitudes on the outcomes of the case.

Preliminary results of the pilot study indicate that females tended to interpret the decision of the Bobbitt case as a positive victory for women, whereas men tended to see this as an anxiety-producing threat toward their future heterosexual relationships. The male–female discussion groups tended to be more guarded in their general attitudes. For example, in the male–male group, many conversations sounded like this: "When we men go to bed, we will not be feeling as safe as we use to.... I can't imagine a life without a dick, a man is not a man without it." In the female–female group, a sample conversation was, "I feel really happy that she was acquitted.... Finally, a woman stood up for herself; abused women have to stand for themselves because men rule this society, and women are always a little meager, a little weak. Finally a woman took matters into her own hands and did what she had to do to break the cycle."

In Buddhism, the notion of "dharma" conveys the principle of correct conduct by the individual. One of the greatest dilemmas of ancient civilizations concerned itself with the rules regarding human behavior and the responsibility of humans to fulfill them. This problem is still facing and fazing our postmodern society, yet it comes with a new twist, considering the fact that our contemporary problems are of a different substance than those of ancient societies. My conclusions here point to the fact that dreams are a major source to help us get in touch with these basic, unresolved problems.

6

Terrorism, Organized Crime, and Social Distress

> It is safer to believe evil of everyone
> until people are found out to be good,
> but that requires a great deal of
> investigation nowadays.
> Oscar Wilde, *A Woman of
> No Importance*

In the aftermath of the bombings of the World Trade Center (WTC) in New York City and the federal building in Oklahoma City, newspapers published maps showing the radius of potential destruction from such blasts. The ballistic results were frightening as were other scenarios concocted about attacks on the vulnerable infrastructure of bridges, subways, buildings, and tunnels.[1]

Three decades ago it would have been inconceivable that several persistent, unresolved ethnic-nationalist conflicts in the Middle East and southwestern Asia, along with a deeply alienated individual, could act in such an unprecedented manner to produce a level of violence resulting in the death and wounding of hundreds of civilians. All of this would have been thought preposterous; but it happened.[2]

With terrorism endemic in several countries and regions—Northern Ireland, Bosnia, Lebanon, Rwanda, Sri Lanka, Peru, India, Somalia, and Liberia—the young have become child warriors. In too many cases violence and armed conflict are a natural part of everyday life for them. Having witnessed numerous car bombings, assassinations, military battles, and atrocities against civilians, many young adolescents and preteens see violence as the only way of handling grievances and problems.[3] For many youths in conflict-ridden areas, there is a desperate need to identify with some type of authority figure who might give their lives some direction and meaning. Unfortunately, the role models often turn out to be terrorists and guerrillas who perpetuate much of the violence. Abu Nidal could attract young people who were poor, with limited educations, who felt betrayed but didn't know why; with little to look forward to, these beknighted youngsters prepared to sacrifice their lives because of the personal gratifications they derived from bonding with such powerful charismatic figures. The brutality of the acts and the cruelty of the perpetrators matter less than the strength the terrorists represent by virtue of their daring and their skills with weapons and the science of killing. They also symbolize authority by means of their presumptive commitments to the cause and its movement toward social, political, economic, cultural, and, most important, psychological liberation. Identifying with the terrorists and joining their commandos are not merely thrilling and adventurous but the logical things to do for many hapless adolescents. Not to become part of it would seem idiosyncratic.

Continuing terror and the emergence of "mustang states" made up of aggrieved minorities bitterly resenting past repression, as in Russia and the former Yugoslavia, pose serious problems. A small group or an emerging state does not need to develop a well-organized military establishment given the power and sophistication of modern weapons, and coercion and extortion on a massive scale are more readily feasible as a negotiating strategy in interstate conflicts. Another aspect of terrorist potential has to do with the rank and file of organizations. They will in all likelihood continue to be filled with the poor, uneducated, and alienated young of the Third World and elsewhere. But as the World Trade Center bombing and Oklahoma City illustrate, the disaffected and disenfranchised may also be joined by extremists who possess technological sophistication and operate in sociocultural and economically retrogressive structures. These are individuals skilled in the modern technologies of the computer, telecommunications equipment, information databases, and financial networks who add a new, frightening repertoire to the primitive terror tactics of the past. Having previously avoided sabotaging telecommunications and financial networks because these lacked melodramatic media effects, and because such operations were technically demanding, contemporary terrorists are now equipped, skilled, and willing to engage targets that have high publicity value. With few exceptions (the Tamil Tigers of Sri Lanka and the Peruvian Shining Path come to mind) terrorists worldwide have stayed within the operational frameworks of proven tactics: bombings of key symbols of authority and repression, kidnappings of elitists, hijackings of innocent civilians for media coverage, and assassinations to spread fear and weaken the resolve to resist. But as the targeted communities of business and government have hardened their security crusts, the terrorists have taken notice.[4] What once seemed too complicated and outrageous to tackle has become more appealing as the tools become available.

HIGH-TECH WEAPONS AND "SMART" TERRORISM

Before the dissolution of the Soviet Union, the possibility of international pirates and terrorists obtaining nuclear weapons seemed no more than an exciting movie script. Now, with the USSR a memory, even the FBI has openly acknowledged the threat of weapons seizures by mafias who could market them to outlaw states.

A disturbing aspect of black-marketing high-tech weapons is the role of Third World nations in all of this. The arming of Third World countries is a trend for which the United States and the former Soviet Union are principally responsible. In the 1980s a brisk trade developed in the selling and supplying of deadly weapons and explosives to guerrilla armies, nationalist liberation struggles, and government military establishments involving many countries in addition to the superpowers: China, India, France, Germany, and other nations were active in the arms markets of the Third World.[5] The prospects of weapons clandestinely finding their way into terrorists' hands cannot be dismissed in the chaotic political climates of so many states. (All extremist groups need is sufficient supplies of cash to obtain what they want.) And this procurement of sophisticated weapons has meant that many extant security measures at airports, embassies, and other places have become obsolete.

In the aftermath of the 1991 Gulf War, a new surge of arms dealing occurred with the demonstrated effectiveness of high-tech weaponry in winning that war. Another factor spurring the sale and transfer of weapons was the restructuring of the balance of power in the Middle East following Iraq's defeat. While the arms trade is organized around national states and not geared specifically toward terrorist groups, the sheer abundance of weapons coupled with the instability of regimes increase the risks that weapons may fall into terrorists' hands.

Of all the ominous trends, the most worrisome is the prospect of terror escalating with the availability of weapons of mass destruction. The collapse of the Soviet Union portends several troubling trends that may actually heighten rather than diminish world tensions. First, many highly trained scientists, engineers, and technical specialists from within the Soviet military-industrial complex may be lured by smaller states eager to build up their own nuclear arsenals. These wandering nuclear "mercenaries" would be relatively easy prey for irresponsible potentates prepared to pay handsomely for their services. Second, there is the serious question of who will control nuclear weapons in the former Soviet Union. Although the former republics initially agreed that nuclear weapons would remain under Russian central control, Ukraine quickly changed its tune and asserted territorial rights over the weapons within its borders. What happens should the Commonwealth of Independent States—the confederated entity succeeding the Soviet Union—disintegrate in the clamor of ethnic-nationalist and religious differences among its many members? It is likely that other states within the brittle structure of the Commonwealth may decide to control—worse, sabotage—nuclear facilities and weapons located within their national boundaries. And should that occur, the prospects for extremist groups gaining possession of such powerful weapons increases exponentially.[6]

To return to the WTC bombing plot, the government made the case that the defendants in the trial (including Sheik Omar Ahmad Ali Abdel Rahman) planned a war of urban terror against the United States. The charges against Rahman and 11 others were that the Trade Center bombing was part of a conspiracy of several attacks planned to disrupt the country. It was alleged that the conspiracy was organized to blow up the United Nations building, FBI headquarters in New York City, and Hudson River tunnels and to assassinate key political leaders in the United States. Had the plot succeeded, the Trade Center attack would have been the beginning of fearsome psychological tribulations and traumas overshadowing the pain and suffering from the physical damage. However, the threats themselves should not mislead us into thinking that a terror campaign necessarily would lead to massive mental breakdowns in the population; such prophecies are not only unscientific but actually harmful in that they can result in apathy and anxiety. Indeed, if the historical evidence from World War II is of any value at all, it suggests that the recovery capabilities of populations tend to mitigate the effects of physical deprivations and psychic distress.

SURROGATE VICTIMIZATION

As important as the physical effects of terrorist bombings, the psychological and social impacts cannot be calculated or measured with the same accuracy. But given that limitation, it is possible to arrive at some reliable estimates. Cities such as New York, Paris, London, or Chicago are complexes of interrelated functions combining both physical and social components. For purposes of analysis, this functional interdependence can be broken down into various homogeneous relationships between social and physical factors. A relationship may be construed as "functionally homogeneous" if it basically serves only one function in a city. For example, housing as a relationship between dwellings and dwellers (rather than a fixed quantitative datum of actual units) is functionally homogeneous because it chiefly serves the one purpose of accommodating city inhabitants. From such physical/social relationships, we can derive generalizations and regularities showing how a city's social functions are affected by different degrees of terrorist destruction. Trends can be extrapolated beyond the range of empirical data from other urban environments to obtain assessments concerning the social effects and ramifications of terrorist attacks.

ELASTIC URBAN RELATIONSHIPS:
POSITIVE AND NEGATIVE RECIPROCITIES

The empirical evidence from World War II along with events over the past three decades in the Middle East, Northern Ireland, Italy, West Germany, France, Turkey, and Indonesia suggest that cities are capable of making adjustments to physical destruction in much the same way as a living organism responds to injury. If a section of a city is attacked and virtually destroyed, the effect is not as if it were merely lopped off. There are compensatory reactions. In New York City, the emergency situation caused by the WTC bombing intensively mobilized and affectively utilized its physical resources more than under normal conditions. The Trade Center bombing showed that a certain amount of physical destruction does not eventuate in an equivalent loss in social functions. The point can be made hypothetically in this way: If, for example, 50 percent of the houses in a city are destroyed (as occurred in the World War II air war over German and Japanese cities), it might still be possible to accommodate the entire population through doubling-up in the remaining intact dwellings. Similarly, a partial loss of transit facilities can be absorbed by crowding more passengers into the remaining rolling stock and vehicles.

These ecological flexibilities of urban populations became apparent in conditions of natural disaster where massive storms, floods, fires, and major geological events like earthquakes disrupt normal functioning. Up to a point the recovery capacities of populations attenuate the destructive physical effects. During World War II, for example, the RAF at night and the American Army Air Corps during the day raided and "wiped out" major German cities, but analyses of the strategic bomb survey data documented that no comparative socioeconomic damage in the area physically erased by bombing raids occurred at first, so that the war potential of the population was not seriously impaired in the short run. Housing losses in Dresden, Hamburg, and other industrial cities did not result initially in either a parallel population loss or a decline in the labor force. In most of the German and Japanese cities exposed to constant air attack, population loss was smaller than housing loss at the beginning stages of the bombing campaigns. However, the cumulative effects of the bombing over time on the physical infrastructure did have a deleterious effect on population and precipitated a decline in industrial output capacity of war materials and an erosion of social order. In sum, after physical destruction exceeded a certain critical percentage of a city's total infrastructural resources in power, transport, housing, and communication, the increase in aerial bombardment resulted in a disproportionately larger increase in negative social effects.[7]

CRIMINALS, TERRORISTS, AND ENTREPRENEURS: OPPORTUNE LINKAGES

Perhaps the global dimensions of terrorism constitute one of several indicators of general psychosocial transformations where personal identities derive from a series of "fragments" rather than coherent social wholes such as class groups, traditional religious orientations, or mainstream political affiliations forged in the Cold War polarities of communism, capitalism, and liberal/conservative ideologies. These "new" cultural and political identities—gender, race, sexual orientation, ethnic, and nationalist—manifest themselves very often as confrontational countercultural challenges to established elite definitions and are themselves in constant agitation, decomposing and recomposing, revealing their inherent instability.[8]

Terrorism as a method of conflict often sheds its originary roots in political struggles. That is to say, terror as a methodology rather than an ideology has emerged as an instrument appropriated and exploited by criminal groups and state entities. Criminal organizations such as the Sicilian mafias and American La Cosa Nostra have historically regarded apolitical terror—the indiscriminate use of violence—as an indispensable instrument in their business enterprises. Within some politically oriented movements, terror is strategy designed to instill general fear, to be sure, but also to provoke a government into mere reckless acts of repression so that the political conflict is sharpened, clarified, and, in effect, simplified.[9] Coincidental with the spectacles of blown-up aircraft, skyscraper explosions, and brazen daylight murders of government officials in South America, Europe, Asia, and Africa is a long, squalid history of state-sponsored death squads and policies where individuals are summarily executed and specific groups systematically exterminated.[10] There is no need to dwell on the well-documented details of terrorist and counterrerrorist atrocities other than to reiterate the point that the distinction between a member of Black September (the 1972

Olympic Games attack against Israeli athletes in Munich) and one who explodes bombs in a commercial location as part of an extortion attempt is a valid one. The behavior of each surely contains significant elements of terror, but does it contribute to our understanding by lumping them together and treating them from the perspective of criminal behavior? The conventional wisdom sees important distinctions between violent acts that are actually criminal events in terms of the motives of the perpetrators. There is no doubt that in many respects terrorism resembles common crime—that, for instance, an aircraft hijacking for the release of political prisoners resembles in all details a hijacking for money.

Nevertheless, in a vital sense the similarities are misleading because the politically motivated hijackers rarely act from purely selfish reasons. Usually, they are members of a political organization that sanctions the act in the name of political goals. Further, the phenomenology of terror is such that a hijacking or a bank robbery would not be an isolated event—as criminal acts tend to be—but part of a medley of actions, criminal in the strict sense, but intended primarily to achieve some political purpose however farfetched. Most important, terrorists involved in criminal activities claim to represent an aggrieved group of some kind and to be acting on its behalf. This is why they do not consider themselves criminals of any kind but revolutionaries, patriots, and (to use that trite term) "freedom fighters." Of course, their announced goals and identities may be utterly unjustified, in which case the crime metaphor seems descriptively accurate and pertinent. But what if, despite appearances to the contrary, a small collection of violent individuals with no visible support from, or endorsement of, a mass movement, act on their own hoping to function as a political vanguard igniting popular resistance. We cannot simply assume that such violence is not related to a mass movement. Claims of representation raise interesting and important questions that should not be decided summarily or by terminological definitions alone: violence-prone groups and the masses they purport to serve politically, even in criminal endeavors, is a matter of motivation. Understandably there is a tendency—especially among the opponents and victims of terror—to see the lofty ambitions of terrorists as mere rationalizations for criminal behavior. The question is how to test the validity of such claims.

The chief defect of the metaphorical assignation of terrorism as crime is its failure to admit the possibility of a continuum linking terrorism and armed struggle to mass political violence. On the one hand, to assert that violence is criminal behavior even in a politically revolutionary context is to decide that it is not integral to a process of political change; on the other hand, to contend that terrorist acts are essentially acts of war even when they are no different behaviorally from criminal actions is to say that they are integral to the political struggle. Disputes organized around these constraining contentions prejudge events and are not really about the meaning and applicability of terrorism to violent events. Actually, terrorism resembles crime and may be criminal behavior, but it also can represent an early phase in a war of liberation or repression. The lines between terrorism and crime are often blurred so that these issues cannot be easily resolved. During the past decade there have been media discussions and reports of the merging of terrorist organizations and drug traffickers conspiring in what has been dubbed "narco-terrorism."[11]

THE "GRAY AREAS" OF CRIME AND TERROR

What appears to have developed in some of the more volatile regions of the Third World, Eastern Europe, and the Mediterranean is an alliance of traditional criminal organizations and political insurgencies (terrorist groups) with corruptible governments. In part, these sinister partnerships may result from an explosive expansion in the international demand for cocaine and other illicit substances that naturally attracts opportunists from the business community, law enforcement, terrorist groups, political parties, and sovereign governments.[12] An interesting geographical aspect in the emergence of narcoterrorism is the proximity of traffickers and terrorists where both inhabit the same regions of political unrest and narcotics production; it is especially notable in the rural sections of Third World nations where government control is weak or nonexistent and where political insurgencies constitute a sort of parallel government reminiscent of mafia control in the hinterlands of Sicily and Calabria. In the Italian setting, Mafia was the government in many provinces and expanded in the decades after World War II to constitute a major challenge to "legitimate" government in Palermo and Rome. Indeed, the legitimacy of the elected legislatures in the provincial and national capitals was dubious given the systemic corruption of politicians, police, military, the banks, and entire sectors of the Italian economy.

I am suggesting that transnational criminal organizations such as the Mafia and Colombian cocaine cartels pose serious threats to the security of their host and home states. As with the Mafia in Italy, the axis of power in Colombia may have tilted in favor of the Medellin and Cali cartels: Their willingness to use force against the state and its law enforcement agencies—captured succinctly in the phrase "silver or lead," meaning accept bribes or die—brazenly challenges the state's monopoly on violence and force and can be more destabilizing than the activities of terrorist groups.[13] The Colombian judiciary has been decimated by assassinations and bombings, and the levels of violence in the streets often reaches levels reminiscent of the civil wars and street fighting in Germany, Kabul, Sarajevo, and Somalia. What happened in Colombia occurred in Italy where the Mafia created an illicit and highly effective authority structure with its own rules, territory, and armed forces. Through wealth earned in heroin trafficking across southwestern Asia, the Mediterranean, and the United States and now with connections in the cocaine trade from Latin America, the Sicilian Mafia has massively corrupted and recklessly murdered to further its aims. In the late 1980s mafiosi killed magistrates, policemen, politicians, civil servants, journalists, businesspeople, trade unionists, and each other and did so with impunity because they had neutralized the dominant Christian Democratic party and compromised government at all levels.[14]

Criminal opportunities in the 1990s have emerged in Eastern Europe and the former Soviet Union. According to Williams[15]:

> There is also evidence that the Colombia Cartels are shipping cocaine through and to Eastern Europe; that opium is being shipped into and through Central Asia from Afghanistan; and that Kazakhstan, Turkmenistan, Uzbekistan, Tajikistan and Kyagyztan are increasingly involved in opium and hashish cultivation. (p. 105)

Equally disquieting is the emergence of major criminal organizations in Russia itself.[16] The collapse of the Soviet regime has meant opportunities for organized crime of all kinds, including racketeering, massive fraud, murder, corruption, and money laundering on an unprecedented scale.

The connections among a variety of criminal organizations and terrorist groups including the Hong Kong Triads, opium cultivators in the Shan states of Myanmar (Burma), and the Golden Triangle is matched by drug organizations in Pakistan that expeditiously move their illicit product through the Balkans and Russia. Other key players include Nigerian criminal groups (which deal mainly in heroin and cocaine) and the vaunted Japanese Yakuza engaging in a varied assortment of organized criminal activities including handling methamphetamine (speed) manufacture and distribution on a worldwide scale.[17]

The end of the Warsaw Pact, an international political event of immense significance for the entire world, has also been a profound benchmark for international crime. Claire Sterling[18] sees the consequences and connections:

> Even before the Soviet Union disintegrated altogether, the Sicilian, American, Colombian, and Asian mafias were hooking up with the Russian underground that circled the globe. All have been growing prodigiously rich since then by swapping their dirty money for Russia's real estate, factories, shops, and above all weapons and raw materials, bought on the cheap and sold for up to a thousand times more abroad.
>
> Russia had a runaway black market, a huge potential for producing and moving drugs, an enormous military arsenal, the world's richest material resources and an insatiable hunger for dollars of whatever provenance. Furthermore, it had a rampant mafia of its own, in need of Western partners to make the most of these prospects. (pp. 14–15)

Liberated Russia has attracted Western lowlife, and its "mafia" looks West toward profitable markets and opportunities.[19] The threat may be real but enforcement agencies are in no position to investigate and have no lawful right to do so, and their Eastern and Russian counterparts lack the laws, resources, personnel, and official commitment to investigate, prosecute, and convict organized criminals with predictable consequences. Russia is now a gigantic racket, a safe haven and bridgehead for international crime syndicates; it is the hungry steppe wolf looking West at the sheep but also at the same time consuming itself. But unlike the Sicilian Mafia, the nebula of professional, organized criminals and illegal entrepreneurs, as Jimmy Carter calls them, has no central coordinating council to provide structural integrity and coherence (no "commission" of top bosses), nor does there seem to be a hierarchical structure of authority—capos, Dons, underbosses, soldiers—as found in the American La Cosa Nostra and some Colombian mafias. Thus there are no structural origin myths about ancestors, bloodlines, or heroic figures that make for historical continuity and cohesion; yet the proliferation of these admittedly ephemeral gangs invade every aspect of life, usurping and corrupting political power, overwhelming the rackets of the old party bosses, engaging in extortion, vice, forgery, currency manipulations, contract murder, arms smuggling, and drug trafficking—all on an increasingly international scale.[20]

Russia and, until quite recently, large parts of Sicily constitute what may be called "gray areas"—regions where control in all of its forms and expressions has shifted from legitimate governments to quasi-political criminal power structures. A good example of the gray areas phenomenon (GAP)—apart from Russia, which is in an institutional degenerative phase—may be found in Central Asia (Afghanistan, northwest Pakistan, Kashmir, some former Soviet republics, and China's Xinjong province), Latin America (Colombia, Ecuador, Bolivia, and Peru), the Middle East (Lebanon), and southern Italy, mainly Sicily.[21] Students of the phenomenon think that the proliferation of GAP occurred over the past decade through mergers of ideologically demobilized guerrillas and terrorists with cartel criminals providing illicit goods and services—mainly drugs. These criminal coalitions are not all new. The end of the Cold War reawakened the underworld and increased its visibility and facilitated its power. It also prompted the reemergence of marginal groups that lay dormant during the Cold War. They include (among others) ethnic factions, religious fundamentalists, militias, terrorists, and local mafias that appear to be developing international alliances and linkages. Usually, these groups typically seek to evade, sometimes undermine, and sometimes act in concert with legitimate governments and at other times—as in the case of the Sicilian mafias and Colombian cocaine cartels—gain significant influence or even autonomous control over parts of nations and their governments. Their criminal activities alone enable them to systematically corrupt and intimidate public and private officials; others effectively defy government sovereignty, while still other groups do not attempt to control geographic territory but manipulate, defraud, and corrupt international systems through money laundering, illegal banking and currency practices, narcotics trafficking, and illegal alien smuggling on a transcontinental scale as in the case of Chinese "snakehead" smuggling syndicates.[22]

What multiplies the effects of these activities are the use of sophisticated information and communication technologies and the brute facts of the increasing global interdependence in almost every sphere of life. Because the potentials for power, wealth, and their accoutrements are so enticingly realizable, groups with disparate motives may be tempted to form regional and transnational alliances of convenience and branch out into new combinations of criminal activity. The resulting threats that GAP poses are not just growing political chaos and anarchy at local, national, and regional levels but challenges to world political economic systems, with potentially dire results not for economic elites per se but for the working classes upon whom they prey. In its current incarnation, GAP as a conceptualization seems, at least, amorphous, lacking the conventional precisions of scientific variables, and for this reason it should be treated as no more than a sensitizing perspective, not as a scientifically validated dependable analytical research protocol. For those working in the field of international organized crime and terrorism, one senses intuitively that GAP as a concept may be too elastic for scientific designs and research regimens even though the idea captures persuasively what seems to be a global pattern of action among criminal and terrorist groups springing to life in those regions of the world in the throes of radical change.

Pax Mafiosa and the Trinitarian State

The historical view that terrorism reflects a special psychological breakdown of moral and legal inhibitions against violence, tends to ignore other distinctive provenient sources whose analysis sets the stage for my argument about the dynamic conditions affecting the restraints, limits, and suspensions of power and force used by, for, and against the state. State claims of unconditional security that is, rationales and justifications for legislatively inundated coer-

cive force in order to preserve itself—are being undermined techno-
logically by economic forces and political upheavals that seem to
have propelled us back to the age of Metternich. It is helpful here not
to exclude the kind of nihilistic violence that occurred in Oklahoma
City because that too is symptomatic of the discontinuities, conflicts,
contradictions, and chaos in the capacities of a state to contain
violence and crime. The horrendous bombing in Oklahoma City
was carried out, apparently, by individuals who feel betrayed and
disaffected on all sides—not least of all by the perceived abuse of
state power where individual rights are capriciously denied and
trumped by government prerogatives.

A literature on what is referred to as the "politics of displace-
ment" is developing that tackles the question of the applicability of
rights and their application. Historically, the Bill of Rights was
understood as legal immunities—guarantees against government
intrusion—that belonged to civic beings, that is, to people rooted in
a network of familial and communal relationships that made up
civil society. This civic notion of rights has now been displaced by
the idea of rights as the entitlements of individuals freed of any and
all ties of reciprocal obligation, mutual interdependence, and responsibility. In this formulation, every issue of private life is interpreted as inherently political, and every public issue is made into an
episode that blurs the private and public realms by an uncom-
promisingly individualist conception of rights that results in a politics of group identity that weakens civic ties.

With the hollowing out of civic life comes the death of public
discourse that occurs when politics becomes no more than encounters of warring identities, as is happening in extreme form in
Yugoslavia, the former Soviet Union, and in milder form in the
United States where the common interests or common ground collectively shared seems to be disappearing. In political cultures
where civility and public life are in decay, where communities are
fractured by the undisputed authority of individual choice and self-
realization, it is possible that no space is left for public debate,
discourse, and the practice of politics.[23] Paradoxically, contrary to
theories of economic determinism, economic prosperity may be
more dependent on healthy civic institutions (as Chomsky has
tirelessly claimed) than on market forces of unfettered capital flows
and investments. If anything, as the late Christopher Lasch has

argued, the free-market enthusiasts have contributed to the prole-
tarianization of the working and middle classes through rising debt,
falling incomes, and unrelenting job insecurity.[24]

With economic enrichment for a corporate elite barely touched
by the caprices of the economy, with technological vitality unabated,
and with communal attachments and civic engagements treated as
optional extras on a fixed menu of individual choice and market
exchange, the ground for vast social dislocation, urban desolation,
and economic stagnation and impoverishment swells and prolif-
erates. In dwelling on the psychological effects of a polarized economy, there is the danger of investing trivial incidents of anger with
the ponderous social or psychological significance of alienation. The
two are so often connected that "alienation" is our inscription for the
impression of continuity and the uninterrupted multitude of hates,
jealousies, and envy that because they are successive innumerable
occurrences—though each is single and ephemeral—creates an illusion of unity out of which the notions of anomie and alienation are
formed.

The right extremists have moved from a posture of rhetorical
reaction to what they perceive as threatening social change symbol-
ized by the changing racial complexion of the country, its ethnic
diversity, and the encroachments of the federal government. The
consequent radicalization of their fear has meant that they have
armed themselves to defend their perceived jeopardized rights and
status. What complicates matters are the available means by which
they resist and defend themselves. What I refer to is weapons
technology and access to it, but I want to avoid the implication that
technology itself is the sole, ultimately determining instance of our
present social distress. Still, as Van Crevald[25] points out, the means
of sophisticated war-making machinery, which was once the province of nation-states, is now available to a wide range of nonstate
players including drug traffickers and terrorists. He writes that, "As
the second millennium A.D. is coming to an end, the state's attempt
to monopolize violence in its own hands is faltering" (p. 192). Moreover, nation-states, such as the United States, often seem muscle-
bound militarily and inflexible when dealing with, or even attempting to understand, GAP issues, organized crime, and terrorism. The
inevitable evolution into chaos that institutional inertia entails can
be witnessed in the Balkans, the former Soviet Union, and else-

where. Ironically, as technology appears to be opening the door to globalism and the accompanying economic and scientific interdependence, tribalism and the re-grouping of people in terms of xenophobia, alienation, and social distress are on the upswing.

Van Crevald[26] offers some observations on the modern conditions of warfare that are pertinent to the issues of crime, violence, and terror. In particular, his notion that "trinitarian warfare—government, the army, and the people" (p. 193), the traditional bedrock of the nation-state system—is on the verge of collapse is a useful concept in the analysis of powerful mafias linked with terrorist groups that are lavishly equipped with modern weapons. The potential for state destructuring, rooted in technology and an ideology of tribalism and functionalism, creates an environment in which violence becomes privatized and is no longer the exclusive domain of the state.[27]

The questions posed at the outset concerning the modern threat of organized crime and terrorism can be approached through a consideration of a country that has lived in agony because of the power accrued by gangsters or terrorists. The best example is Sicily. Since the beginning of the century, Sicily has lived in the shadow of the Mafia, which has persisted through fascist, socialist, and democratic political regimes; it has accordingly neutralized the powerful Roman Catholic Church and compromised law enforcement from central to provincial governments.

Over the past 25 years, the Mafia utterly terrorized Sicilian society and helped to bring the first Italian Republic close to collapse through the carefully planned murder of judges, senior police officers, and recalcitrant politicians. Witnesses knowing the reputation of mafiosi for "omerta"—the law of silence—would hesitate to provide incriminating evidence that could be marshaled to pursue a prosecution. Through bribery and threats, the Mafia also established a virtual monopoly over public works, making the costs of roads, hospitals, office buildings, and multiple-dwelling apartment buildings four or five times the free-market price. Protection money is a regular unofficial tax paid to the underworld by practically everyone involved in commerce or industry. Small wonder then that private outside investment dried up and some northern Italians now believe that their political union with this island should be severed because of its criminal liabilities.

There are probably no more than 6,000 "men of honor"—as mafiosi still refer to themselves, even though any honorable aspects of their behavior are buried in the past—and perhaps another 100,000 people dependent on them for a livelihood. The Cosa Nostra has managed to entrap a population of 10 million in its criminal clutches by colluding shrewdly with successive governments of all ideological persuasions thereby guaranteeing its immunity from prosecution. What has unraveled the Mafia in its modern incarnation is its unbridled greed: the influx of vast sums of money from its brilliantly orchestrated international drug trafficking produced fierce infighting among the "families"; hundreds were assassinated, especially among the leading Palermo cosche (groups). The new, victorious "Boss of Bosses," Salvatore (Toto) Riina from Coreleone, used methods that resembled those of the Colombian narcoterrorists: massive bombings in which innocents were killed, and other cruel and barbaric methods of murder became commonplace. Because of his viciousness, few assassins were captured, even fewer convicted, and it was obvious that witnesses and magistrates were bribed or simply intimidated by the savagery—a Sicilian version of the Colombian "lead or silver."

Over time, however, public opinion was emboldened against the Mafia by the confluence of events that could not be anticipated, and because these circumstances were fortuitous the fact that the Mafia has been checked should be seen optimistically but cautiously. Methods for effectively coping with modern, transitional organized crime groups are still formative and evolving. Success is temporary and arguably exaggerated; for example, the brutal murders in 1992 of the leading prosecutors, Falcone and Borsellino, coincided with larger momentous events that weakened the protective shield the Mafia has assiduously cultivated for decades: the dominant Christian Democratic party. With the disappearance of the Italian communist party in 1990, the Christian Democrats could no longer tout themselves as the bulwark against a Red revolution that the Red Brigades a decade earlier portended. And with the end of the Cold War, Sicilians were better able to see the Mafia—far from defending Sicilian interests—as colluding with Roman, southern, and foreign interests to keep the island backward.

Events since the nationwide investigations, arrests, and convictions are, however, not particularly encouraging, with many Mafia leaders in hiding and much of their huge wealth transferred to legitimate businesses that are hard to identify. If nothing else, the Mafia learns from its misfortunes. It is active internationally with a reputation unsullied by setbacks in its homeland. Its major new projects may involve the refinement of its structure to sharpen its organizational mobility in an age of transnational, high-tech business and crime. The Mafia's future strength is not only its nomadic freedom but its flexible, versatile institutional structure, its chameleonlike capacities. It is a great crime and war machine: vicious, clever, aggressive, and now more and more transgressive.

The evidence of widespread social distress as indicated by community collapse and economic stagnation in places like Palermo, Moscow, and Bogota begs the question: Will it not be one of history's cruel surprises if Palermo and Moscow represent the future of Washington?

CONCLUSIONS

With the collapse of the former Soviet Union in 1991, the fine line separating political, paramilitary, and criminal elements in the republics has often been blurred. In August 1995, that disturbing fact of juntas, corrupt politicians, and a confused, ambivalent public was reinforced by an assassination attempt against Eduard Shevardnadze, the former foreign minister of the USSR and now a leading candidate for the presidency of the Georgian parliament. Fortunately, Shevardnadze survived, barely. The damage and injuries were a warning: In the center of the capital city, Tbilsi, the motorcade went up with a bomb and the initial reaction was that the attack had been mounted by a radical, dissident political terrorist group, but it quickly became evident that the local Georgian mafia orchestrated the incident. Shevardnadze was expected to win the presidential elections scheduled in November, and he had promised to eradicate organized crime, which he described as the most serious destabilizing force in the entire Transcaucasus region.

The incident illustrates the convergence of two phenomena that historically have been separated in public consciousness primarily because the official machineries of political and criminal justice defined them as different in motivations and purposes. But terrorism and organized crime are kindred processes. With their uncanny capacities to correctly identify the sensitive political pressure points that yield concessions, or that will produce accommodations and compromises, they are capable of neutralizing through astute corruption strategies and intimidation the oppositional forces arrayed against them. As a methodology, terrorist violence is not particularly unique to politics or politically inspired revolutionary change; organized crime groups have utilized bombs, kidnappings, and assassinations as organizational assets—indeed, violence in its myriad forms was and is an integral part of organized crime groups everywhere.

The distinction between the two, between organized crime and terrorism, cannot be mounted on the type of violence associated with each activity, nor can it depend upon criminal behaviors; groups usually are distinguished and differentiated by their motivations and goals officially defined and described as either terrorist or mafia. While we do not wish to discredit the validity of this distinction, the realities are that organized crime groups and terrorist organizations are often intertwined, adopting each other's tactics, personnel, and operational styles. Thus, to say that terrorists function from moral high ground however appalling their practices, and that mafias pursue an agenda of personal greed and self-aggrandizement, is to ignore the empirical evidence suggesting that the interactive effects and suffusions of tactics, methods, personnel—the intermingling of organizations, in short—profoundly affects their goals and identities.

The attack on Shevardnadze serves as a prism for weighing our thesis that what is at stake in the post–Cold War era is not merely institutional decline and the systemic erosion of institutions resulting in massive social distress, but that the political cultures themselves are incapable of adapting to new circumstances; this lack of a coherent set of values and normative constraints means that little stands in the way of incipient anarchistic social forces (organized crime and terror) from spreading. Another question implied by the first is whether the acceleration of terrorism and organized crime is indicative of continuing institutional paralysis and fragmentation. I think it is. However, this issue is far too large and complex to be explored in depth here. What may be said is that the clarification of the problems will not be helped by "simplification" through a mass media whose time and space for such things are circumscribed by what Chomsky refers to as organizational "concision" in the presentation, articulation, and dissemination of news. Sound bites are, after all, sound bites, not arguments, perspectives, theories, points of view. In the milieu of mass media, conventional pieties masquerade as reasoned conclusions and positions. It is well to remind ourselves that the raison d'être of media is chiefly to make money and secure audiences, and only secondarily to inform. And it is also well to keep in mind that many structural forces are at work that do not facilitate the reformulation of problems whose breadth and scope are extraordinary. For example, in the United States and elsewhere, there are powerful escapist dogmas and practices (religious fundamentalisms, drugs) at work that inhibit the exploration of new approaches to problem solving. More importantly, perhaps, are the lingering sociopolitical divisions and separations of national boundaries and jurisdictions that may have been geographically and strategically appropriate a century ago, but are irrelevant today.

The bipolar (or tripolar) world of East, West, and North/South (Third World) is disappearing as new embryonic coalitions and configurations of states supplant the old alliances. Within these orbits of power, everyone is obliged to grapple with the challenges of crime and violence stretching across continents involving the shifting pace and changing locales of economic growth and stagnation: technological innovation on an unprecedented scale in environments that are dangerously brittle with ethnic and racial minority feuds. Despite this, the evidence warrants some optimism, contrary to the prevailing gloom: We are comfortable with the strategic theorem that says that no general set of rules provides decision makers with morally and ethnically informed courses of action that may be universally applicable (which may explain the consistent failure of the UN in Africa, the Middle East, Latin America, Asia). The central challenge is to face up to collective social distress that seeps through entire societies like a virus. How it can be understood and defined is a chief task for psychosocial analysis.

Finally, we are more sanguine than Rieff, for instance, who concludes his study of Freud with the pessimistic observation that the character ideals that formed Western culture and energized it— political man, economic man, religious man—no longer dominate Western civilization. For him, "psychological man," Freud's contribution, replaces the archaic stereotypes of the past. Psychological man seems angst-ridden, withdrawn, cynical, and deluded, repudiating the optimism of the rationalist Enlightenment, retreating deeper into the self, convinced that the intellectual legacies of the past are no more than irrelevant burdens in a world incapable of transforming itself.

Ironically, the West may not have failed at all but managed (in spite of itself) to transport along with its treachery, violence, and guns its cultural imagery and conceptualizations during the imperialist era. All of the characterological traits Rieff thinks have been abandoned may be operative today on a global scale. The entrepreneurial spirit is like a plot flung into space that pervades Asia; the pressures toward political democratization are also evident worldwide. Lifton points out agreeably that we (contrary to the rather rigid, Gotterdamerung image that Rieff portrays) are protean, and why suppose that others living in different cultural worlds and experiences are not also protean and capable of change, flexibility, and vibrancy. I will further elaborate on this point in the concluding chapter.

Being "Good" in "Bad" Places

Toward a Principled American Lifestyle

> Congress shall make no law, says the First Amendment.
> I need make no comment, says the Fifth Amendment.
> Who, then, shall take responsibility to let right be done?
> The experts say the people must minister to themselves,
> While all goes down before us.
>
> R. W. RIEBER

> Memory, false or otherwise, captures our phenomenology of time.
> Does the clock record time, or create it?
> Neither. It just pulsates the rhythm of our mind.
>
> R. W. RIEBER

The point of view that I have advocated throughout my analysis of the social distress of our times may be perceived by some to have certain irrefutably cynical overtones. In describing given psychosocial problems, I may seem to have reached some rather pessimistic conclusions. These might lead the reader to consider my evaluation of the current state of affairs to be a skeptical outlook, with bleak and dismal possibilities for the future.

Ambrose Bierce's definition of cynicism classifies it as "a defect of vision causing the subject to see the world as it really is rather than as it ought to be." In keeping with this attitude, the major objective of my exploration of the psychopathy of everyday life initially consisted in taking a careful look around to see what is really going on rather than to desire to evolve a panacea. I did not seek to provide a formula or theory to palliate the social distress that I described, nor did I try to find a cure for the psychosocial virus causing society's dysfunction. My method was to scrutinize and analyze the prob-

161

lems of our society. At this point, however, it is necessary to consider some means of action that the average citizen could take against the social distress and psychopathy of everyday life. We must collaborate to take concerted action to move our society toward a principled lifestyle in which the values that contribute to social distress will not dominate our thinking and our behavior. The worst thing to settle for is a quick fix. Quick solutions frequently create more problems than they solve. The technology that developed "the Club" to prevent car theft might, in fact, stimulate the invention of new and better modes of thievery in order to circumvent the quick fix.

If in the midst of darkness there exists light, then in the midst of light there must also exist darkness. The mind exists in both light and darkness, and, under certain circumstances, darkness illuminates the mind with more clarity than light itself. Having examined the dark side of society and having become acquainted with it makes it easier to consider possible ways out of the darkness. This is a journey that will lead us, eventually, to help design the foundations of a more enlightened society.

PRINCIPIA AMERICANA

The national character of the United States is held together by a thin thread of crazy glue. The special components linking such a heterogenous mass of conflicting concerns, interests, and values are a puzzle that will always mesmerize social scientists.[1] Such conflicting elements obscure our ability to find a secure place and role in this society. This heterogenous structure, taking its most evident shape in the inner cities, represents perhaps the most crucial object of exploration.

What specifically can bind such inconsistency into a stable pattern? What consistency must our crazy glue have? The answer to such a question would undoubtedly provide the information necessary to create a meaningful whole out of our society's dysfunctional fragmentation.

From the understanding gained of the causes of social distress, through the descriptive analysis of the psychopathy of everyday life, the assertion can be made that the most substantial binding force is the integrity of the institutions out of which society's cultural structures are built. Institutions in every society must be sturdy and capable of withstanding the pressure by certain marginal groups operating dysfunctionally. We saw in Chapter 5, while attempting to understand the nature of societal distress, that without the integrity of social institutions, the linking thread is in terrible danger of being torn apart. It becomes necessary to stress the importance of understanding the significance of the malignancy growing in the fundamental institutions of our society—the family,[2] the educational system, the religious system, the government—as a first step toward reconstruction.

In order to better understand the evolution of American materialism, let us now briefly summarize the historical background of the American Dream. As a social, economic, and political ideal, as a daydream about a self-sufficient egalitarian democracy, it has been a pivotal point in shaping the American mind. This utopian vision arose from the very important framework of equal opportunity developed by our Founding Fathers. Accordingly, the democratic ideology has played an important part not only in the political but also in the social and economic development of the United States— and currently influences and shapes the roles of many other nations on this planet. This democratic ideology affirms that all individuals have *the right to participate in shaping their lives and destinies.*

This persuasive assertion grew primarily out of the integral design of the democratic government of the United States. It was emphasized during the Civil War period, and presumed to extend itself during the Industrial Revolution as a function of capitalism. The premise that all citizens may participate actively in the design of their modus vivendi contributed greatly to the development of both science and technology. An individual breaking new ground with a given invention or discovery that might promote the general welfare or improve the common defense became an object of respect and praise from the nation as a whole.

A second point of importance in the development of our national character involves the philosophy of individualism, which grew out of the minds of the great thinkers of the Golden Age of American literature—the brainchild of authors such as Henry David Thoreau and Ralph Waldo Emerson. Every individual in the society has *the capacity to change for the better in accordance with his or her needs and desires*, and the man who does not march in step perhaps "hears a different drummer."

This individualism became a capitalistic philosophical ideal that was represented in the "do-it-yourself" principle, as evidenced in the children's story about the little red hen who plants the seeds, reaps the harvest, grinds the grains, prepares the dough, and bakes the bread, all by herself, with no help from any of the other animals. When the bread is ready to eat, the others ask her to share it with them, but she declines, just as they had refused to share the work with her. Though such behavior might seem rather arbitrary and capricious, when it becomes directed toward the benefit of the society such a serious attitude—embracing a feeling of pride in one's individual work and endeavors—plays an important role in the improvement and advancement of not only the individual but also the group. After all, the other animals learned a very good lesson: if they wanted to eat, they had better begin considering working for their meals.

The American national character emerged from the standards of both equal opportunity and individualism. The "American Dream," tarnished as it may be, has not yet been replaced by anything else. Despite evident belligerence in distressful psychosocial circumstances, Americans still subscribe to these premises and have inculcated them in their children through the decades by means of four crucial institutions: the family, the school, the church, and the government.

The family embodies the first and foremost provider of rudimentary discipline and moral training, while also imparting the knowledge and skills required to adapt to the adult society. This institution has the task of creating a microsociety for the child by supplying the necessary emotional security, along with the more complicated obligation of bestowing upon the child the fundamental rules for functioning in everyday life.

The process of growth that the child undergoes under the auspices of the family is intertwined with the development of the child during his or her years in school. As its major objective, the school aims to institutionalize the child's mind to the greatest possible extent, so that the child may follow a prescribed image of life— life as it ought to be led. Education in this country has always been given one of the highest priorities in the process of cultivating both the body and the mind. Ideally, the educational system trains and enhances all the various aspects of human existence, including reason, the affections, the imagination, aesthetics, literary and scientific skills, and so forth. In a holistic, integrated scheme of values, in our potentially enlightened society, education could (but doesn't) represent in and of itself, in terms of its methods and teaching programs, an indispensable part of the natural order of things.

The institution of the Church, with its formal, organized religious lifestyle in the context of our pluralistic society, in accordance with the ethical arguments of our founders, has furnished some important particularities for the development of the national character. Following the philosophical principles derived from the ideas of William Paley and John Locke, one can identify the Church's most important task as the instillment of morality and a stern ethical code. Sectarian differences ought not to represent an overwhelming hurdle, since they should be tolerated in the spirit of mutual respect.

According to the founders of this nation, the Deity is to be appreciated not only through the study of the scriptures but also through an accurate study of nature, the work of the Creator. This attitude, brought to America in rudimentary form by the Puritans and remaining alive in some measure to the present day, provides for the connection between a belief in both the value of the individual's inner life and the importance of self-knowledge.

Questions relating to time and the cosmos are partitioned into two subdivisions: historical criticism and scientific investigation. One may view the role of the American national character as an ideal that has been formed through a process of curing the soul through the hand of God (religion) and curing the mind through the hand of science (psychology). The Church can invest these functions of morality, namely history and science, with a certain degree of sanctity while additionally supporting the state that makes its own survival and proliferation possible. Ultimately, the doctrinal differences varying from a given church to another constitute an insignificant and trivial matter.

Let us turn our attention now to the functions of the government as a disseminator of values. The popularity of the image of the self-made man led to the character development of the self-made American who could do everything and anything. That was originally the image of the American farmer, an outgrowth of the rugged individualism of the pioneers who settled the West and developed the agrarian movement. However, small, rugged, individualistic farming families in this country are becoming obsolete as the interests of big agrarian capitalism become more successful in remaining profitable.

Gradually this ideology, the image of the self-made man, is becoming undermined by the very financial, governmental, and religious systems it supported. In part, such an outcome is the result of the full development of the Protestant tradition in the United States, which has been motivated by two main trends: natural religion and millenialism. The naturalists saw God not only through scriptural revelation but through the accurate study of nature or creation reflecting its Creator. This intense interest in nature amounted in some cases to virtual deification of nature, driving God out of the picture and reflecting science as its major prophet.

The second trend, millenialism, expressed God through acts of humanity. These acts were to lead to the perfection of humanity through consistent, rapid, and rational progress. The intermixing of religious, political, and scientific psychological trends led to such psychopolitical-religious concepts as "manifest destiny" and "might makes right," soon becoming defacto theology in all large modern states. Patriotism gradually replaced the God that the study of nature was undermining. Natural religion took its psychological cues from science by declaring that "the proper study of mankind is man." This new understanding, with theological overtones, was to be applied toward the gradual improvement and redemption of humanity.

Insidiously, humanity has come to be regarded primarily as "masses" and individualism itself was mutating into "mass individualism." The most effective way to "cure" humanity was through the combined effort of perfected social and political institutions with the possibility of constructing a perfected society. The "American Dream" was certainly turning out to resemble a new recipe for the landscaping of yet another utopia, a never-never land of sorts, where the principles of equal opportunity and individualism were quickly fading as the control of mass culture became the first priority of social and political institutions.

Furthermore, let us not forget the role of the media in terms of mind pollution. Based on their perception of their own interests, the media define one of their major roles as a kind of "spin doctor" whose responsibility is to diagnose the state of the mind of the people in general, and the social institutions in particular.

Consequently, they carry out this mission by taking the pulse and temperature of the nation in order to inform it of its present condition—"a self-fulfilling prophecy" as it were. The rationale for all of the work is that the media are providing society with what it wants and needs. Eventually this so-called service takes on a life of its own both for the spin doctors and their patients. The people learn to need and feed upon this manufactured entertainment as if it were real. The result for consumers becomes a prepackaged construction of their own reality. The more they need this merchandise, the more they believe it, and the more they believe it, the more they need it. In the final analysis a socially patterned defective media addiction sets in and the people are hooked, booked, and cooked.[3]

We have seen how the four institutions of the family, the school, the church, and the government are the primary components bound together by the peculiar crazy glue we mentioned earlier. The Founding Fathers proclaimed that "all men are created equal" and that they are endowed by their Creator with certain unalienable Rights, that among these are Life, Liberty, and the pursuit of Happiness.

From the time of the Declaration of Independence to the present day, however, these inalienable rights may or may not have been secured by the institutions created for that purpose, and we have witnessed a gradual degeneration of those institutions. As we observed in more detail in earlier chapters, the malignant web of the psychopathy of everyday life has spread throughout our valued institutions, having spawned a virulent disease at all levels of the contemporary scene. The question to address now concerns the reaction of the individuals of our times to this phenomenon.

Homo Mutabilis

Proteus was the son of the Greek god of the sea and the keeper of his father's army of vile and atrocious sea monsters. Mortals came to him to ask questions about their futures, as he had the marvelous power to foresee events. Proteus also possessed the ability to metamorphose into any form he wished and had quite a knack for mutating into wonderful and terrifying shapes that would scare away the innocent humans who went to consult him. Robert Jay Lifton describes the individuals of our times as *protean men*—men exploring change, men capable of shifting allegiances, loyalties, and principles to suit the times, and men of distorted ethical codes overburdened with conflicting values.[4]

Lifton makes an attempt to understand the problems of post-modern individuals and their society by introducing the term "self-process," i.e., the individual's understanding of the self as a symbol of his or her own psychological organism. "The self-process," explains Lifton, "refers to continuous psychic recreation of that symbol that represents an internal and external exchange process." He contends that a new style of self-process is emerging everywhere, "a new understanding of the self" that primarily "derives from three factors responsible for human behavior."

The first factor is "the psychobiological potential common to all mankind at any moment in time," in effect, our inherited capabilities; the second emphasizes the socially inherited cultural traditions into which we are born; and the third are those traits that arise from the contemporary historical courses occurring during our lifetimes. That which is contemporary history makes up an important part of the self-process and is frequently in conflict with the part arising from cultural tradition.

"Psychohistorical dislocation" is caused by a break in the sense of connection that humanity has long felt in the vital and nourishing symbols of culture—family, idea systems, religions, and the life cycle. At the same time that they are carried internally, they are considered burdensome. The self-process appears to be an attempt—sometimes constructive, sometimes destructive—to find alternatives.

Lifton also attributes the emergence of the protean man to a flooding of imagery resulting from an extraordinary flow of post-modern cultural influences over the mass communication networks. This overabundance of information, crossing regularly over local and national borders, deters the protean man from committing himself to a single form while, at the same time, intensifying his need to practice a protean style of self-process.

Protean man, freeing himself from an institutionalized self, also severs ties with the classic superego and is, in an object-relation sense, fatherless. Therefore, his dependency needs are not met and he becomes suspicious and disdainful of all apparently nurturing institutions, even those he reaches out to. Fearful of counterfeit nurturance, he derides the very institutions of commerce, academia, or service to a cause from which he seeks nurturance, and in the death of the classic superego gives birth to the concept of "the neo-Capitalist hero." (Incidentally, Ross Perot is probably the best example today of the power of this image.)

Protean man, in the course of self-process, overturns all and secretly feels guilty for having no symbolic structures to carry his loyalties and his achievements. Feeling abandoned by those same institutions, fear and anger are his responses to appropriate targets. Still longing for the nurturance and stability he despises, he will join extremist sects and political movements, court violence for a just cause—no matter how temporary—to try to empower himself with money, sex, cars, and drugs.

"The central impairment here is that of symbolic immortality," says Lifton,

> of the universal need for imagery of connection predating and extend-
> ing beyond the individual life span, whether the idiom of this immor-
> tality is biological (living on through children and grandchildren),
> theological (through a life after death), natural (in nature itself which
> outlasts all) or creative (through what man makes and does).

Lifton has further developed his theory of self-process in two later works, *Self* and *The Broken Connection*, in which he extends his description of the disintegration of the self. According to this later elaboration, the self is not the intrapsychic entity accounted for in the traditional psycho-dynamic approach. Instead, Lifton here envisions the self as a dialectic, dynamic process of interaction between various levels of society and the individual. Stress is the major contributor to the disintegration process between the components of that dialectic.

In individual psychology, to lose oneself provides an opportunity to find oneself. The same logic can be applied to the societal level: If a society loses itself, that is, it malfunctions to the point that it feels lost—a point to which our postmodern society certainly has arrived—then this very same society has an opportunity to develop a way to find itself again and it may aim to proceed in a different and more promising direction. From this perspective, one can clearly see the parallels between Lifton's visualization of the self-process, my interpretation and explanation of social distress, and the psychopathy of everyday life.

Looking for a Marketplace for Wisdom

In these tempestuous times, when the quality of life supersedes in comfort and luxury that of any other earlier period due to our most advanced science and technology, we are faced with some quite complicated options for living.

Individuals living in the last quarter of the twentieth century can choose alternative familial setups, alternative styles of education, alternative formal or informal faiths, and alternative norms for societal organization. Clifford Geertz[5] states the problem as follows:

> The world is a various place, various between lawyers and anthropologists, various between Muslims and Hindus, various between little traditions and great, various between colonial thens and nationalist nows; and much is to be gained scientifically and otherwise by confronting that grand actuality rather than wishing it away in a haze of forceless generalities and false comforts. (p. 234)

It is time to take some clues from all the above. To face the problems caused by such diversity and conflicting value systems involves picking certain codes and rejecting others. In one certainly valid option, as Huxley provocatively suggests in the preface to *Brave New World*, "You pays your money and you takes your choice."

The question is how to simplify the plethora of options and to boil them down to a sensible few. If we take the central set of problems to be *the deprivation of mankind's options and the disempowerment of his participation in satisfaction of his needs by authoritarian symbolic structures*, whether that be within family, education, religion, or the workplace, then there is obviously a better way.

How then do we generate that self-correction before our social and individual excesses reach the breaking point?[6] In a way, protean man and his self-process mode of functioning is an attempt to restore a homeostatic balance by rejecting the bankrupt, false values of a pseudodemocratic capitalist society. Society needs to give credibility to this process of self-creation. Constructive support of the self-process can also restore mankind to his innate psychic need for symbolic interests through returning in a new way to family, theology, nature, and creativity. The way to support the constructive aspects of the self-process is by engaging his increased participation and encouraging his efforts in producing desirable changes in the rejected, currently unsatisfactory social structures—in the family, education, religion, and the workplace. It means trusting that the need for survival and symbolic immortality are powerful enough to enable him to override the destructiveness of the fear and anger generated by his alienation from himself and his society. Active participation in his education, in his psychological and medical treatment program, in his spiritual development, in family activities and concerns, in the way productivity occurs in the workplace—all will help return a sense of balance and connection between the individual and society. The society must be prepared to have many of its traditional modus operandi questioned and changed and in that sense become a self-process kind of society. Only by acknowledging and absorbing pragmatic, humanistic values will a true democracy be restored, not just politically but in every aspect of social interaction.

We can, on the one hand, opt for a highly materialistic and dehumanizing way of life, thus maintaining ourselves adjusted to the Western ideal, leaning toward easy rewards of financial abundance while we continue to deny the existence of all the skeletons in our cultural closet. On the other hand, having understood and accepted the nature of our problems, we can turn ourselves and our mores around and redesign our life cycle by favoring the important aspects of humanistic interdependence and basing our actions on participation, sincerity, respect, and responsibility.

The American culture has always been prepared to believe in the truth until it finds out what it really is. Our challenge as individuals and as a society is to become courageous without being reckless, to become ethical without being self-righteous, to become wise without being cunning, to become responsible without being alienated from purposeful action.[7]

As we approach the twenty-first century, there is a critical mass of perceptions that recognize the problems and demand changes in the way that the government has been overseeing social institutions. This demand for change is part of the self-process of the larger social conscience. Among these changes is the recognition that a more active participation on the part of the individual is a prerequisite for healthier economic, educational, and familial institutions.

Participation also becomes the key word that underlies the "women's choice" movement. It is not simply the statement that women have the right to an abortion, but that they have rights as individuals to participate in the society in their own particular ways, ways that are organismic as well as psychological and social.

There seems little question that governmental policies for the past decade have brought at least an earlier condition of homeostasis to a critical danger point. For instance, the foreign and domestic policies of the Reagan–Bush administrations offered the philosophy that might be summed up as follows. When you do it, make sure you do it secretly. Then be careful to cover up its illegality in order to claim that it has the highest morality. The information offered by the survival-oriented motivations of the society at large have been influencing the political body to reassess its attitudes. The feedback from the dehomeostatic state of the individual, as evidenced in the declining economic, educational, psychical, and mental health of the nation, has caused demands for changes. Feedback from the workplace and its economic statistics causes demands for changes in the economic systems; feedback from the schools shows that decline in intellectual accomplishment is endemic enough to endanger other social institutions, especially the capitalistic workplace; feedback from health care shows expanding costs as well as expanding sickness; feedback from planetary ecology reveals a threat of disaster that makes necessary changes in the governmental regulation of capitalist and societal modes of operating. But can and will the governmental and judicial systems effectively, not cynically, carry out their critical regulatory roles in monitoring the changes that are called for?

Active participation, individual choices, and freedom to make medical as well as psychological and religious decisions imply an enhancement of the potential that exists in our society for new individual commitments. Insofar as the need for the freedom to make decisions was cynically bypassed by those persons adopting or adapting to the psychopathy of everyday life, there was a moral retrogression contaminating every aspect of social behavior. The public's violent reaction to the Rodney King decision in Los Angeles was prompted by its lack of trust not only in the Los Angeles Police Department, but in the criminal justice system as a whole. The individuals who took over the streets setting fires, looting, and hurting people reacted also to their lack of trust in the decision of the jury—perceived as supporting an intolerable status quo. The public then went on to do what has seldom been done: to judge the jury, manifesting their discontent with the judicial system and with American government as a whole. People in Los Angeles rioted when they became frightened, as well as angry, because the institutions providing for the general welfare were failing to work for the benefit of the people.

The reaction in Los Angeles to the Rodney King verdict is just another shadow of the zeitgeist of postmodern America. More recently, the reaction to the decision to the Simpson case throughout the world is a further example of a similar process in the postmodern era. One interpretation of the above is that the jury system itself is on trial. It resurrects the motto hanging on the wall of the barbershop (in Melville's novel *Confidence Man*) of the showboat Fidele, "No Trust." The messages related to it still remain with us. If we are to build something useful, we have to build trustworthy institutions. The inability to trust is part of the inability to love—a very dangerous frustration that turns itself into self-hatred. Hatred turned inward turns into psychophysiological illness and ultimately into hatred turned outward. This situation constitutes a great and present societal danger that was manifested in the King debacle.

The investigative analysis of the psychopathy of everyday life has been an attempt to take the first step toward resolving the constantly growing web of social distress inherent in contemporary society. We have seen that the problem, because it is endemic, has been generating awareness of the need for changes in the levels of individual social participation. Our goal must be to increase the national democracy, and the national responsibility and conscience, by increasing the opportunities for choices and participation in every institution upon which America is founded.

In this discussion, I have provided some preliminary broad strokes that describe the way toward a principled, more responsible, and freer lifestyle. I have argued that the root causes for the rise in psychopathy and social distress are to be found in the progressive ruptures in the system linking the individual to the social group via a system of shared values. We cannot afford to ignore these ruptures; not only will they continue to make trouble, but they will make even more trouble when they operate out of awareness. And recognizing them is not enough; we must begin repairing them. Normalized psychopathy in high places, in my view, is largely the result of social distress as it has become institutionalized in the emerging world culture. Put simply, the psychopathy of everyday life will continue to prevail until we cease to be proud of those things of which we should be ashamed.

NOTES

PREFACE

1. E. Fromm, *The Sane Society* (New York: Bantam Books, 1956).
2. A. Kardiner, *The Individual and His Society* New York: Columbia University Press, 1939).
3. G. Bateson, *Mind and Nature: A Necessary Unity* (New York: Dutton, 1972).
4. R. W. Rieber and M. Green, "The Psychopathy of Everyday Life: Antisocial Behavior and Social Distress," in R. W. Rieber (Ed.), *The Individual, Communication, and Society* (New York: Cambridge University Press, 1989).
5. R. W. Rieber and R. J. Kelly, "Substance and Shadow: Images of the Enemy," in R. W. Rieber (Ed.), *The Psychology of War and Peace: The Image of the Enemy* (New York: Plenum, 1991).
6. R. J. Kelly and R. W. Rieber, "Psycho-Social Impacts of Terrorism and Organized Crime: The Counter Finality Partico-Inert," *Journal of Social Distress and Homelessness*, 4(4):265–286.

INTRODUCTION

1. Many authors have written about the steady decline and disintegration of family life in America in the last 50 years; C. Zimmerman's book *The Family of Tomorrow: The Cultural Crisis and the Way Out* (New York: Harper Brothers, 1949) is one of the best on this subject.
2. The 1993–1994 international political arena seems to illustrate that world culture has slowly but surely assimilated and incorporated the psychopathy of everyday life in many ways. For example, a number of prime ministers have been forced to resign in Europe, and over half of the politicians in Italy are in the process of being brought up on charges of various forms of illegal activities. The political situation in Brazil is somewhat more complex in that the political corruption is so widespread and institutionalized that most experts feel that, at least in the near future, popular exposure of this problem and change are very unlikely.

175

3. An interesting article by Edward Iwata describes serial killer Ted Bundy's character as well as his tendency to engage in what I have chosen to call "the manipulation of meaning in the communication of deceit." See E. Iwata, "The Baffling Normality of Serial Murderers," *San Francisco Chronicle*, May 5, 1984.
4. Steven Cohen, professor of Russian Studies at Princeton University, has called attention to the fact that with the collapse of the Soviet Union the probability of a nuclear accident is even more of a problem than it was under the Soviets because we have more than one government or agency to deal with plus the possibility that they may sell to others.

CHAPTER 1

1. H. S. Sullivan, *Interpersonal Theory of Psychiatry* (New York: Norton, 1953).
2. J. B. Calhoun, "Population Density and Social Pathology," *Scientific American*, 206(2):139–146 (1962).
3. C. Turnbull, *The Mountain People* (New York: Simon and Schuster, 1972).
4. L. J. West, "The Psychobiology of Racial Violence," *Archives of General Psychology*, 16(6):645–651 (1967).
5. A. Kardiner, *Individual and Society* (New York: Columbia University Press, 1939).
6. Ibid.
7. G. Wallace, *The Great Society: A Psychological Analysis* (New York: Macmillan, 1914).
8. T. Veblen, *The Theory of the Leisure Class* (London: Macmillan, 1899).
9. Kardiner, *Individual and Society*.
10. E. Fromm, *The Sane Society* (New York: Reinhart, 1956).
11. The notion of the family should include both male and female relationships. In today's culture we seem to find ourselves in a house rather than a home, somewhere between *Brave New World* and *1984*. The home has gone the way of the mental health system; sometimes it appears to be a madhouse, sometimes a halfway house, and sometimes (with the homeless problem) an outhouse.

P. Tolan's findings indicate that "... a family's ability to support each other and to harness that support to cope with transitions and stress during adolescence relates to a lower level of antisocial behavior." Tolan mentions four types of social stressors that can be differentiated by the level and manner of impact that they have on the individual's psychological adjustment:

1. Traumatic events
2. Daily hassles
3. Induced transitions
4. Developmental transitions

When looking at antisocial behavior, no given stressor alone can account for antisocial or delinquent behavior. The interaction of these factors as a process is the most profitable method of coming up with a fruitful explanation for this problem. P. Tolan, "Socioeconomic, Family and Social Stress Correlates of

Adolescent, Antisocial and Delinquent Behavior," *Journal of Abnormal Child Psychology* 16(3):317–331 (1988).

Berger and Berger discuss the problems of the family in relating to the society at large. They succinctly put the matter as follows: "The problem was not maladjusted individuals or social groups but rather the sick society, of which the sick family was an integral part" (p. 16). B. Berger and P. Berger, *The War over the Family: Capturing the Middle Ground* (Garden City: Anchor Press Doubleday, 1983).

12. Etzioni's work on communitarianism, as well as his previous research, provides ample documented evidence for this problem. A. Etzioni, *Communitarianism* (New York: Crown, 1994).

13. "The Family: Home Sweet Home," *The Economist*, September 9, 1995, 21–25.

14. Kant, in one of his lesser-known works, *Anthropologie in Pragmatischer Hinsicht* (Section 56, Frankfurt 1798), makes the following observation of the character type of a certain class of people whom we have identified on a continuum or spectrum from psychopaths all the way to "the psychopathy of everyday life":

But one guild of these so-called men of genius (better, monkeys of genius) is placed under this shop sign; they speak the language of minds extraordinarily favoured by Nature, declare laborious learning and research to be dull-minded, and profess to have seized the spirit of all science at one clutch, and to dispense it in small doses, concentrated and strong. This race, cousins of the quacks and criers at fairs, is very prejudicial to progress in scientific and moral culture. They pronounce in decisive tones upon religion, politics and morals, as if they were illuminated and adepts, envoys from the throne of wisdom, while the secret object all the time is to conceal the real poverty of their minds. What else is there to be done but to laugh and continue patiently at our industry, without regard to those mountebacks?

It is interesting to note that Kant's recommendation regarding this matter is not to take these people seriously; this is something that could have been done much easier during the latter part of the eighteenth century, in contrast to the twentieth or twenty-first century with its mass media and high technology. Today it is dangerous not to watch and study this condition carefully. Nevertheless, too much attention, especially in terms of media coverage, is a good illustration of this problem.

15. Ringer describes the problem with great precision.

In sum, the frontiersman and pioneer were bearers of a bifurcated value system. In their relations with their fellow whites, they positively valued things that are deemed virtues in human society; in their relations with Native Americans, they positively valued things that are generally deemed vices in human society. [Frederick Jackson] Turner failed to capture this paradox of the frontier. The very experience that he contended was instrumental in the development of democracy and individualism on the frontier was also instrumental in the development of racism and a racist orientation toward the Native American. This duality is the central meaning of the frontier heritage in America.

In the final analysis the multiculturists have raised a number of fundamental questions and issues about America's paradoxical past, problematic present and uncertain future. These merit serious consideration and will require reexamination of some of the basic assumptions and premises upon which established scholarship has been built. The danger is that such a scrutiny will deteriorate into verbal warfare more frequently associated with an emotional conflict over sacred dogma than a scholarly debate over competing historical interpretations and premises. (B. Ringer, *We the People and Others*, [New York: Rutledge, 1992])

16. It is of some importance to recognize that even such a prominent scholar as Griesinger, who was a leading force in the transition from the early nineteenth-century school of romantic psychiatric thought to the late nineteenth-century medical/biological paradigm, was cognizant of what we have defined as social distress, despite the fact that this concept was largely underdeveloped during his era. Furthermore, it should be also be noted that the period during which Griesinger was writing of was one of rapid social change. The middle part of the nineteenth century spawned the Industrial Revolution, which with its emphasis on manufacturing and big business produced big changes in people's lifestyles throughout the world. Although these developments of the past are not comparable to the high information-processing technologies of today, the parallels with regard to the manifestation of social distress are still quite strong. For example, Griesinger says,

I would rather coincide with the opinion of most medical psychologists, that the increase of insanity in recent times is real, and quite in accordance with the relations of modern society, in which certain causes, according to experience, exerting a great influence, which cannot however be quite expressed in figures, have become stronger and more extended. The progress of industry, art and science necessitates a general increase of the cerebral functions; the constantly increasing departure from simple modes of life, and extension of the more refined mental and physical enjoyments, bring with them desires and emotions formerly unknown. The general possession of a liberal education awakens in the minds of many a feeling of ambition which few only can gratify, and which brings to the majority but bitter deception. Industrial, political and social agitations work destructively on individuals, as they do on the masses; all live faster—a feverish pursuit of gain and pleasure, and great discussions upon political and social questions, keep the world in constant commotion. We may say, with Guislain, that the present state of society in Europe and America keeps up a general half-intoxicating state of cerebral irritation which is far removed from a natural and healthy condition, and must predispose to mental disorder: thus many become insane. The demoralising influence of large towns—in Paris it is estimated that there are 63,000 individuals who maintain themselves by dishonest means and at the cost of society, in London there are thousands of children already devoted to crime and prostitution—the greater frequency of celibacy, the altered relations of religion, may be considered as co-operating circumstances ...

For further information see W. Griesinger, *Mental Pathology and Therapeutics*, translated from the German (2nd ed.) by C. Lockhart Robertson and James Rutherford (London: New Sydenham Society, 1867).

17. Leonard Saxe's hypothesis concerning the ubiquitous nature of lying is clearly compatible with the point we are making. For example, Saxe says,

although discussion of public figures found to have lied makes it appear that deceitfulness is a disease that afflicts solely the rich and powerful, the correlation is spurious. In some cases, public figures are spurious because of their lies; in other cases, their renown obscures the universality of deceptiveness. From individuals who lie to a partner about their other intimate relationships, to students (and professors) who create excuses for late papers, to salesmen and lawyers for whom deceptiveness can be a normatively sanctioned aspect of their daily work life, the lack of truthfulness is too common to be restricted to those who make headlines ... if the hypothesis about the universality of lying is correct, something pernicious has occurred; along with other social problems, we have defiled our interpersonal relationships. Paradoxically, this seems to have become a society in which lying is endemic, but in which a Victorianlike attitude is also maintained that heavily sanctions those who are caught in prevarication. (p. 412)

See L. Saxe, "Lying: Thoughts of an Applied Social Psychologist," *American Psychologist*, 46(4):409–415 (1991).

18. Another variation on the theme of a clandestine international arms sale can be seen in the International Signal and Control (ISC) affair. Initially created and supervised by the National Security Council and later by the Central Intelligence Agency, the ISC was discovered to be selling armament parts through its South African branch to Middle Eastern countries for exorbitant profits. It was later ascertained that the president of ISC, Jamie Garson, sold the company to an English firm for 1.4 billion dollars, despite the fact that the actual market value of ISC was substantially lower. Consequently, the English firm went bankrupt because it found itself unable to meet the financial obligations of its stockholders, which left Garson as the sole reaper of profits. Ironically, all of this occurred under the "watchful" eye of CIA deputy director Robert Rayamond, who is up for confirmation to become a Cabinet member.

19. In discussing the Oliver North scandal, Saxe (L. Saxe, "Lying: Thoughts of an Applied Social Psychologist," *American Psychologist*, 46[4]: 409–415) makes a pertinent observation that incorporates what we have called the psychopathy of everyday life. For example, Saxe says,

That lies are all around us does not mean we accept lying. To the contrary, the insidious nature of lying seems all too apparent. We are barraged, almost daily, by reports of yet another public figure who has been charged with some form of malfeasance or convicted of a criminal activity. In virtually all cases, these individuals deny the allegations. From political figures such as Mayor Barry of Washington ... to military officers such as Colonel North and Admiral Poindexter ... to sports heroes including runner Ben Johnson ... and baseball player Pete Rose, lying is rife. (p. 412)

20. B. Latane and J. Darley, *The Unresponsive Bystander and Why Doesn't He Help?* (New York: Appleton Century Crofts, 1970).
21. A good example of the psychopathy of everyday life is an incident that took place as early as the 1950s. It was a game show scandal in which major networks artificially created the illusion of intelligence by providing the contestants of a TV quiz show with the answers ahead of time. The suspense built up and these shows became so popular that everyone watched them as if they were about to win the money themselves. Every network developed a show along the same pattern; they even got a psychologist from Columbia University, Charles Van Doren, to take part in the scam. The whole con exploded when one of the contestants provided conclusive evidence to a grand jury that was called in New York State to investigate the problem. During the investigation as many as 200 people purged themselves in the presence of a grand jury about their participation in the affair. (See Frontline documentary on PBS, 1992, which documents the entire affair with interviews with the actual participants).
22. The facts about Milken are as follows: He's a yuppie, middle-class Jew from Brooklyn who went through the countercultural revolution of the sixties and then goes to work on Wall Street. Being a clever, ambitious entrepreneur, he observes that Wall Street and its leaders are all WASPS, excluding the hyphenated Americans and all members of the club. He decides to make the leaders of Wall Street his primary target. He builds up a network of allies consisting of successful business people including all the hyphenated Americans such as the most successful black, Jewish, and Italian businessman who were capable of rising to the top at Wall Street and Madison Avenue. He convinces them—as a successful and profitable and knowledgeable Wall Street broker and entrepreneur—that he can make them a lot of money, and shake up the Wall Street establishment's discrimination against outsiders. In order to achieve this he successfully markets junk bonds, which yield high interest rates but have little substantive value behind them. He has the charisma and salesmanship to convince everyone to back him and he will make them a pile of money. The game plan is to challenge the ruling class. He uses inside trading and price fixing and forced takeovers as a technique to break the Wall Street establishment's leadership. He investigates and finds out which CEO's are in financial difficulty and guilty of mismanaging their own firms. Their security is ensured by picking their own boards of directors, who approve anything they wish. The stockholders are losing money and the firms are in financial difficulty. Enough people (including charities) made money so that his reputation as a reliable businessman was ensured.

Milken's objective was to hit them at their most vulnerable spot; buyout, takeover tactics were his modis operandi, and when he was successful in taking them over he would eventually break the firm up and let it deteriorate while he pocketed his profits and went on to the next mark. Lots of jobs and lots of money were lost because of the Milken operation. But this did not matter since he and a small number of key people make a large fortune.

Al Capone and the Mafia did the same thing in the thirties. The only difference was that Milken didn't murder anyone. He kept it strictly within the realm of financial killing. He used the same methods—namely public relations and charity—as a means of gaining the trust and confidence of many prominent people. He established what amounted to a hyphenated-American mafia to destroy the WASP leadership in big business. Trump and Robert Maxwell were both variations on the same theme but were not a part of Milken's operation and had different objectives.

A PBS Frontline documentary, which told the story of Milken's scam, also contained testimony of prominent individuals Milken had made money for. These testimonies were in support of Milken as "one of the greatest humanitarians of our time," thus cooling the mark out.

23. G. Partridge, *Proceedings of the American Psychiatric Association: First Colloquium on Personality Investigation* (New York: Privately printed, 1928).
24. R. Niebuhr, *Moral Man and Immoral Society: A Study in Ethics and Politics* (New York: Scribners, 1960).
25. R. Lifton, *The Nazi Doctors: Medical Killing and the Psychology of Genocide* (New York: Basic Books, 1986).
26. O. H. Mower *The Crisis in Psychiatry and Religion* (New York: Van Nostrand, 1961).
27. D. Bakan, *Sigmund Freud in the Jewish Mystical Tradition* (New York: Van Nostrand, 1958).
28. R. LaPiere, *The Freudian Ethic* (New York: Random House, 1959).
29. D. Regier et al., "One-Month Prevalence of Mental Disorders in the United States," *Archives of General Psychiatry*, 45:977–985 (1988).
30. C. Ratner, "Concretizing the Concept of Social Stress," *Journal of Social Distress and the Homeless*, 1(1):7–22 (1992).
31. C. Smith-Rosenberg, "The Hysterical Woman: Sex Roles and Role Conflict in 19th Century America," *Social Research*, 39:652–678 (1972).
32. W. R. Grove et al., "Adult Sex Roles in Mental Illness," *American Journal of Sociology*, 78:812–835 (1973).
33. R. Kessler, "Stress, Social Status, and Psychological Distress," *Journal of Health and Social Behavior*, 20:259–272 (1979).
34. B. Wheaton, "The Sociogenesis of Psychological Disorder: An Attributional Theory," *Journal of Health and Social Behavior*, 21:100–124 (1980).
35. J. McLeod and R. Kessler, "Socioeconomic Status Differences in Vulnerability to Undesirable Life Events," *Journal of Health and Social Behavior*, 31:162–172 (1990).
36. Ratner, "Concretizing the Concept of Social Stress."
37. A. Sameroff, R. Seifer., and R. Barocas, "Impact of Parental Psychopathology: Diagnosis, Severity, or Social Status Effects?" *Infant Mental Health Journal*, 4:236–249 (1983).
38. A. Seeman, "Alienation Studies," *Annual Review of Sociology*, 1:91–124 (1975).

CHAPTER 2

1. I discovered this quote, which was written in Morton Prince's own hand in a book I purchased (Morton Prince, *The Dissociation of a Personality*, 2nd edition:

Longmans, 1908) some years ago. The original copy remains in my personal collection.

2. Since psychopaths have developed an extraordinary capacity to act as if they were perfectly normal, i.e., sane, they must be skilled in a cunning manner to dissociate any real guilt that they should feel about their antisocial behavior. If they fail to dissociate they would then be forced to face the guilt as most ordinary people would. In this sense they lack the common decency to go crazy, for that's what they would do if they felt the guilt.

3. It may be of some value to clarify the historical background of the use of the term psychopath. The tendency to view moral failure as illness, instead of as sin or as an expression of some evil principle inherent in the universe, is scarcely new in the Western world. The ancient Greeks considered that certain kinds of behavior, either antisocial or else not in the individual's self-interest, were plainly caused by forces outside the individual. Homer, in the eighth-century B.C., portrayed humans as subject to the whims of the gods; the gods acted upon humans by affecting their feeling center, or thymus, which was thought to reside under the sternum more or less in the area of the thymus gland. The Homeric formula for describing rash, ill-considered, or antisocial behavior typically had it that this or that god put madness in one's breast; alternatively, it was said that Zeus, or whoever, had taken away one's understanding.

Some twenty-seven hundred years later, in 1809, Pinel introduced the term "insanity sans delire," subsequently taken up by Morel (B. Morel, *Traite des degenerescences physiques, intellectuelles et morales de l'espece humaine et des causes qui produisent ces varietes maladives* [Paris, London, New York: Hachette [1857]) to indicate an illness affecting the moral part of one's being. As a classificatory term, "insanity without delirium" opened the way first for "psychopathy" then "sociopathy" and more recently "antisocial personality" as means of indicating an illness of the moral part of one's being that was largely manifested by behavior injurious to fellow humans, though, as a matter of fact, Pinel applied his term to cases that today would be diagnosed as forms of bipolar affective disorder, or manic-depressive insanity. It fell to the Englishman James Pritchard (J. Pritchard, *Treatise on Insanity and Other Disorders Affecting the Mind* [Philadelphia: Caley and Hall, 1837]), who was a disciple of Pinel's, to be the first to describe a more circumscribed kind of disorder that he termed "moral insanity": "madness, consisting in a morbid perversion of the natural feelings, affections, inclinations, temper habit, moral disposition, and natural impulses, without any remarkable [i.e., observable] disorder or defect of the intellect or knowing and reasoning faculties, and particularly without any insane illusions or hallucinations" (p. 16).

Walker and McCuble (N. Walker, and S. McCuble, "From Moral Insanity to Psychopathy, in *Crime and Insanity in England* [London: University of Edinburgh Press, 1972]) have been able to trace the history of the notion of moral insanity from Pritchard's term all the way to the early twentieth-century term "psychopathy." As it happened, Pritchard's (J. Pritchard, *Different Forms of Insanity in Relation to Jurisprudence* [London: Hippolyte Baidliere, 1842]) case histories almost without exception ascribed the onset of the disorder to a specific illness or traumatic event. But among Pritchard's contemporaries and his immediate successors within English psychiatry, the term "moral" was delimited by the exclusion of any kind of physical injury, organic disease, or other physical factors as contributory causes. Thus "moral" came to refer specifically to the emotional aspects of insanity and "moral insanity" to serious mental disorders not characterized by hallucinations, delusions, or manifest disorders of thinking.

On the continent, however, Griesinger (W. Griesinger, *Mental Pathology and Therapeutics* [London: New Sydenham Society, 1867]) borrowed Pritchard's term and used it to designate and describe a group of retarded patients, whom Griesinger termed "weak minded" and who were prone to mischievous, cruel, thieving, and drunken criminal behavior. Griesinger supposed these traits to be hereditary in nature. Under the influence of Henry Maudsley, this notion subsequently came to play a role in the legislation of the Royal Commission on the Care and Control of the Feeble Minded, which in 1913 described "moral imbeciles" as "persons who from an early age display some permanent mental defect coupled with strong vicious or criminal propensities and on which punishment has had little or no effect" (Walker and McCuble, "From Moral Insanity to Psychopathy"). In 1927, further legislation was passed in which "moral imbecility" was redefined as obtaining "In whose case there exists mental defectiveness coupled with strongly vicious or criminal propensities and who require care, supervision and control for the protection of others" (Walker and McCuble).

The significance of this redefinition is twofold: The ineffectiveness of punishment has been dropped as a criterion, and there is no reference to any kind of treatment as potentially effective. Nonetheless, the term was not to be applied in cases that failed to show any limitation of intelligence, even though there might otherwise be an utter lack of any kind of inhibition, restraint, or other evidence of conscience with regard to criminal behavior. The accepted nosological system had thus developed a striking lacuna with regard to nonimbecilic moral insanity.

It was in this general context that the German psychiatrist J. Koch, in *Die Psychopraktischen Minder-wertizbeiern*, Ravensburg: Maier (1891) introduced the term "constitutional psychopathic inferiority." Koch's term covered not only instances of criminality not covered under "moral imbecility" but also neurasthenia, compulsions, impulse disorders, and sexual perversions. For a considerable period of time thereafter, the term "psychopathic" continued to refer to a wide range of nonpsychotic disorders. Indeed, minus the implication of heredity causation, and minus, too, the group now known as psychopaths, the term had roughly the same wide range as did the term that succeeded it and that has itself only lately been abandoned—"neurotic."

It is not altogether clear just when "psychopathic" was first used to refer *exclusively* to antisocial behavior, though it is clear that this usage came gradually into medical currency during the end of the nineteenth century and the early part of the twentieth. There is some evidence to suggest that in at least one American city, Boston, the gradual delimitation of the term was part and parcel of changing modes of state-sponsored mental health intervention. Specifically, as social workers came to be widely employed as agents of social control in the first decade of the new century, the term "psychopathic" became a diagnostic warrant for forcibly hospitalizing two groups of "patients" considered to be socially deviant: single working women who were promiscuous and inadequate men who shunned work. Thus did Koch's term come to be applied, at least in Boston, predominantly to social deviants.

In the United States generally, psychiatric interest in criminals received its greatest impetus from the comprehensive investigations of Bernard Glueck and his associates. Nonetheless, it is David Henderson, a Scottish disciple of Adolf Meyer, who is generally credited with establishing the modern concept of the psychopath in both European and American psychiatry. Henderson's (D. Henderson, *Psychopaths* [New York: Simon and Schuster, 1939]) diagnostic scheme divided psychopaths into three subgroups: (1) a predominantly aggressive type (redolent in many respects of Pinel's concept of moral insanity as well as of Koch's and Kraepelin's concepts of psychopathic inferiority); (2) a predominantly inadequate type, which include liars, swindlers, assorted petty criminals, and the like; and (3) a predominantly creative type. (This last group derived from the theories of Lombroso and Moebius, theories widely popularized by the writer Max Nordau that saw genius and great artistic ability as symptoms of hereditary degeneration and thus as prima facie evidence of disordered cerebral functioning. The hallmark of genius in this scheme was the reliance on certain runaway thoughts or inclinations that were unimpeded by the ordinary inhibitions imposed by common sense, decency, and moral judgment.)

Unlike some of his predecessors, Henderson elected to make his notion of psychopathy purely behavioral; the diagnosis neither excluded nor entailed the existence of contributory organic factors. In this spirit, he described a number of electroencephalographic studies showing a high frequency of brain abnormalities in his aggressive subtype. This led to a very heated legal debate, since the possibility arose that a diagnosis of psychopathy, with or without a correlative finding of brain abnormality, might be used to establish a defense of diminished responsibility. Generally speaking, in the English courts, a diagnosis of psychopathy did gradually win status as potentially part of an acceptable defense, though the chance of winning an acquittal on this basis remained extremely low.

In the United States in this century, the term "psychopath" gradually fell into diagnostic disfavor on the basis of the opinion, held by Harry Stack Sullivan among others, that the psychology was expressed predominantly in the individual's social relations. As Sullivan (H. S. Sullivan, *Conceptions of Modern Psychiatry* [New York: Norton, 1953]) saw it, such persons exhibited a massive incapacity to profit from social experience. Accordingly, beginning in the late 1920s, the term was gradually replaced by the seemingly more precise "sociopath" in the official nomenclature, though among the general public the more vivid "psychopath" still prevails as the term in general currency. "Psychopath" has entered the common language as an epithet with which to deride the moral fiber of one's enemies or people one dislikes. It is used now in legal, professional, and academic circles, as well as by the general public, to refer pejoratively to those who care only about advancing their own material interests and who are willing to do whatever they can get away with. In the most recent revamping of the standard diagnostic system, meanwhile, "sociopath" has yielded to the term "antisocial personality." In part, "sociopath" fell because of its intrinsic relation to the term that it was meant to supersede; insofar as "sociopath" was following "psychopath" into common currency to cover a wide spectrum of behavior, it was no longer suitable for the psychiatric nomenclature.

4. The emphasis of the DSM-IV antisocial personality disorder (APD) diagnosis on behavioral factors that reflect low socioeconomic status may underinclude certain individuals (e.g., white-collar criminals) who possess the psychological characteristics of the psychopath but not the behavioral characteristics of the APD. Cleckley (H. Cleckley, *The Mask of Sanity* [St. Louis: Mosby, 1976]) devised 16 characteristics of the psychopath that putatively are reflected in the characteristics described in the DSM-II. However, the individual classifiable as psychopathic according to Cleckley's criteria may or may not be diagnosed as an APD under the DSM-IV criteria. His criteria are as follows.

1. Superficial charm and good intelligence
2. Absence of delusions and other signs of irrational thinking
3. Absence of nervousness or psychoneurotic manifestations
4. Unreliability
5. Untruthfulness and insincerity
6. Lack of remorse or shame
7. Inadequately motivated antisocial behavior
8. Poor judgment and failure to learn by experience
9. Pathological egocentricity and incapacity for love
10. General poverty in major affective reactions
11. Specific loss of insight
12. Unresponsiveness in general interpersonal relations
13. Fantastic and uninviting behavior with drink and sometimes without
14. Suicide rarely carried out
15. Sex life is impersonal, trivial, and poorly integrated
16. Failure to follow any life plan

5. At the turn of the century, Sidis was clearly aware of the institutionalized greed of the American culture when he advocated the following with regard to the education of children:

The most central, the most crucial part of the education of man's genius is the knowledge, the recognition of evil in all its protean forms and innumerable disguises, intellectual, aesthetic and moral; such as fallacies, sophisms, ugliness, deformity, prejudice, superstition, vice, and depravity.

See B. Sidis, *Philistine and Genius* (New York: Moffat Yard and Company, 1911).

6. Ekman, in a very important book on the psychosocial aspects of lying, discusses

the difficulties in recognizing the deceptive liar. See P. Ekman, *Telling Lies: Clues to Deceit in the Marketplace, Politics and Marriage* (New York, Norton, 1985) p. 57.

7. Bundy is a good example of a psychopath who succeeded for a long period of time without being caught. After he was caught he successfully used the media for his own purposes. We will discuss this further in Chapter 5.

8. H. S. Sullivan, *Interpersonal Theory of Psychiatry* (New York: Norton, 1953).

9. R. D. Hare, "Psychopathy and Sensitivity to Adrenalin," *Journal of Abnormal Psychology*, 79:138–147 (1972); R. D. Hare, *Psychophysiological Studies of Psychopathy*, in D. C. Fowles (Ed.), *Clinical Applications of Psychophysiobiology* (New York: Columbia University Press, 1975), pp. 77–105; R. D. Hare, "Electrodermal and Cardiovascular Correlates of Psychopathy," in R. D. Hare and D. Schalling (Eds.)., *Psychopathic Behavior: Approaches to Research* (Chichester, England: Wiley, 1978), pp. 107–143; R. D. Hare and D. Craigen, "Psychopathy and Physiological Activity in a Mixed-Motive Game Situation," *Psychophysiology*, 11:197–206 (1974).

10. Hare (R. D. Hare, "20 Years of Experience with the Cleckley Psychopath," in W. H. Reid, D. Dorr, J. I. Walker, and J. W. Bonner (Eds.), *Unmasking the Psychopath* [New York: Norton, 1986], pp. 3–27) has created a checklist for assessing psychopathy in criminals using institutional records and personal interviews. Hare has reported high reliability both for a scale consisting of Cleckley's 16 criteria (alpha = .80) and for a scale derived from the Cleckley criteria (alpha = .89) consisting of 20 items. Hare's (1986) 20 criteria for psychopathy are as follows:

1. Glibness/superficial charm
2. Grandiose sense of self-worth
3. Need for stimulation/proneness to boredom
4. Pathological lying
5. Conning/manipulative
6. Lack of remorse or guilt
7. Shallow affect
8. Callous/lack of empathy
9. Parasitic lifestyles
10. Poor behavioral controls
11. Promiscuous sexual behavior
12. Early behavior problems
13. Lack of realistic, long-term goals
14. Impulsivity
15. Irresponsibility
16. Failure to accept responsibility for own actions
17. Many short-term marital relationships
18. Juvenile delinquency
19. Revocation of conditional release
20. Criminal versatility

Hare reports that clinical-behavioral measures, such as the *DSM-III* criteria and his checklist, are more reliable than self-report inventories in the assessment of psychopathy. He reports the following coefficient alphas for self-report scales that are widely used to assess psychopathy.

1. An experimental Self Report Scale based on his checklist (alpha = .80)
2. The Socialization (So) Scale from the California Psychological Inventory (alpha = .73)
3. The Psychopathic Deviant (Pd) Scale of the MMPI (alpha = .65)
4. The Hypomania (Ma) Scale of the MMPI (alpha = .67)

Overall, the clinical behavioral measures and the self-report measures are not highly correlated and form two factors in principal components factor analysis. The two forms of measurement lead to differential diagnoses that create practical and theoretical problems. Many subjects who may be characterized as psychopathic on a psychological basis (e.g., according to the Cleckley criteria) may escape *DSM-III* diagnoses. Similarly, many of those who are diagnosed as psychopathic (i.e., APDs) by the exclusively behavioral *DSM-III* criteria may not be psychopathic in a psychological sense. Hare believes that the advantage of his checklist over the *DSM-III* criteria is that the checklist includes both psychological and behavioral characteristics.

11. Quay (H. C. Quay, "Psychopathic Personality as a Pathological Stimulation Seeker," *American Journal of Psychiatry*, 122:180–183 [1965]) has postulated that psychopathy is based on a pathological stimulation seeking that is physiologically based and that disturbs socialization. The organically based hyperactivity of the psychopathic child causes his or her parents to reject him or her and to impose inconsistent discipline, leading to inferior socialization. Also, the organically based inability of the child to anticipate punishment leads to excessive punishment to which the child becomes habituated, causing him or her to be rejected by others and thereby impairing his or her socialization. Behavioral and psychometric evidence supports Quay's view of the psychopath as an individual in a state of aversive stimulus deprivation that compels him or her to perform antisocial behavior that raises his or her arousal to an acceptable level. However, physiological evidence that psychopaths have either low basal autonomic and cortical reactivity or a high rate of habituation has not been conclusive. The rejection of the psychopath as a child has been strongly supported by McCord (W. McCord, *The Psychopath and Milieu Therapy* [New York: Free Press, 1982]) and the role of emotional underreactivity has received qualified support (D. M. Doren, *Understanding and Treating the Psychopath* [New York: Wiley, 1987]).

Quay's theory has not received much criticism. However, Doren states that Quay's theory is not comprehensive because it does not address the psychopath's absence of guilt, impoverished sense of morality, specific loss of insight, and inability to form meaningful interpersonal relations. Smith observes that the concept of stimulation has been inconsistently defined in research assessing Quay's model. Further, Doren notes that the basis of the psychopath's stimulation seeking has been ambiguously defined in terms of cognitive and affective physiological substrata.

12. H. Cleckley, *The Mask of Sanity* (St. Louis: Mosby, 1976).

13. Although we have used Cleckley's term "semantic dementia" to describe such language, we only adhere to Cleckley's definition in spirit, rather than literally as to what he meant by the concept. We take this term to imply a much richer and broader level of interpersonal communication, implying by "semantic dementia" something more along the lines of a manipulation of meaning in the communication of the psychopath, which amounts to a communication of deceit and deception. Unlike other examples of abnormal language that we have examined throughout this text, it is not the language itself that is deviant. Rather, the aberration lies in the deceptive quality of the language, a language that deceives not only the listener but also the speaker. This language is a tangible and analyzable trait showing the personality or the psychology keeping the psychopath from having the common decency to go crazy. By warping reality to deceive others, the psychopath also deceives himself and in so doing is actually dissociating any feeling of guilt about his antisocial behavior.

   Another example of semantic dementia: Charles Manson, in a recent documentary program on public television, commented while discussing his past criminal behavior, "I don't break the law; I make the law." See Cleckley, *The Mask of Sanity*.

14. Doren (D. M. Doren, *Understanding and Treating the Psychopath* [New York: Wiley, 1987]) has integrated into a theoretical model the theories of Gough (H. G. Gough, "A Sociological Theory of Psychopathy," *American Journal of Sociology*, 53:359–366 [1948]), Eysenck (H. J. Eysenck, *Crime and Personality* [London: Routledge and Kegan Paul, 1977]), Quay (H. C. Quay, "Psychopathic Personality as a Pathological Stimulation Seeker," *American Journal of Psychiatry*, 122:180–183 [1965]), and Hare (R. D. Hare, *Psychopathy: Theory and Research* [New York: Wiley, [1970]). Doren bases his model on his observation that psychopaths are challenged by exerting control over others and avoiding others' control over them. According to Doren's model, the conditioning that produces partial learned helplessness in psychopaths' socialization interacts with their innately low level of cortical arousal to produce a pathological attempt to obtain control over their environment. Partial learned helplessness is produced by a conditioning process characterized by erratic discipline in which the individual is alternately rewarded and punished for the same behavior on an unpredictable basis. This process described by Doren is similar to Bateson's "double bind." Psychopathy may be produced as a result of this type of conditioning in interaction with certain innate dispositions, such as the attention deficit disorder of the "hyperactive" child.

   The low cortical arousal of the psychopath leads to excessive stimulation seeking and to an inability to inhibit behavior that evokes punishment. The behavior emanating from the psychopath leads to erratic discipline that produces partial learned helplessness. The psychopath therefore has fewer socializing experiences and is persistently challenged to exert control over the rewards dispensed by his or her environment. Reward and punishment that are inconsistent and unpredictable force the psychopath to focus on the expectancy of reward rather than the expectancy of punishment in order to avoid complete helplessness. Psychopaths' learned helplessness enhances both their insensitivity to their punishment and their tendency to persevere until their goal is attained. This perseverance results in a limited repertoire of instrumental behaviors.

Psychopaths focus their attention on short-term goals and diminish attention to other details of their environment as a result of both their excessive stimulation seeking and their insensitivity to punishment. Specifically, psychopaths manifest a diminished concern for the negative consequences of their behavior and a narrow focus of attention on stimulating goals. Thus, other people are perceived by psychopaths as obstacles to be manipulated so that they can establish the control over their environment with which they are compulsively preoccupied.

Doren states that psychopaths' absence of guilt, inability to form intimate relations, lack of responsibility, specific loss of insight, and low anxiety and depression are due to their view of both others and themselves as objects of manipulation. However, Doren does not explain exactly how the psychopath's instrumental orientation creates these deficiencies in the psychopath. For example, Doren tautologically states that the psychopath does not feel guilty about hurting others in the act of manipulating them because he or she derives so much satisfaction from the manipulation of others.

15. Gough's (H. G. Gough, "A Sociological Theory of Psychopathy," *American Journal of Sociology*, 53:359–366 [1948]) socialization theory of psychopathy is based on the symbolic interactionism of G. H. Mead. Gough has postulated that psychopathic individuals are incapable of taking the role of the generalized other and therefore lack empathic understanding of the behavior of others. As a result, psychopathic individuals fail to internalize social norms and values, and act without consideration of the effects of their behavior on others. Gough's Socialization Scale is a reliable and valid predictor of delinquency and criminality and has been demonstrated to predict accurate interpersonal perception in experimental contexts. However, only one study has demonstrated that the scale predicts psychopathy, as defined by Cleckley, rather than criminality. Hare has criticized the inability of Gough's theory to explain the etiology of psychopathy, and Smith has criticized the theory as being ambiguous and connotative in its terms and constructs.

16. The disinhibition of antisocial behavior and the creation of a depersonalized state by a deindividualizing situation may be greater in the psychopath who is innately disposed to dissociation than in those normals and psychopaths not disposed to dissociation. The psychopath may be especially disposed either to absorption in the positive affective experience created by deindividuation or to dissociation from the aversive aspects of deindividuation. A deindividuated state permits the psychopath to extend control over others without fear or guilt. However, a deindividuated state may also threaten his or her ability to extend control over others. The depersonalized psychopath given to deindividuation may experience a loss of control that he or she experiences as aversive and that leads him or her to extend pathological control over others. The normal assertion of individuality in response to the negative aspects of deindividuation may be limited in the psychopath to this pathological extension of control over others to obtain rewards and increase his or her deficient level of arousal.

Anomie is defined as a retreatist detachment and despair associated with a sense of contradiction and ambiguity in norms and values that impairs the integration of society (L. Srole, T. S. Langner, S. T. Michael, M. D. Opler, and T. C. Rennie, *Mental Health in the Metropolis: The Midtown Manhattan Study, Vol. 1* [New York: McGraw-Hill, 1962]); Merton (R. Merton, *Social Theory and Social Structure* [New York: Free Press, 1968]); (R. Merton, "Three Fragments from a Sociologist's Notebooks," *The Annual Review of Sociology*, 13:8–10 [1987]) has theorized that deviant behavior is the result of a type of anomie that involves an acceptance of cultural goals and a rejection of the methods approved by society for obtaining these goals. Merton's model of anomie proposes a number of types of anomie based on the acceptance and rejection of cultural goals and methods. The other types of anomie may also be related to psychopathic attitudes and behavior that are diffused throughout the society but which do not necessarily constitute in individuals an APD.

1. *Retreatism*, which involves a rejection of cultural methods but not cultural goals.
2. *Innovation*, or deviance, which involves a rejection both of cultural goals and methods.
3. *Ritualism*, which involves a rejection of goals but a passive resignation to cultural methods.
4. *Rebellion*, which involves a rejection both of cultural goals and methods as well as an acceptance of alternative cultural goals and methods.
5. *Conformity*, which involves an acceptance of cultural goals and methods.

As certain cultural goals (e.g., financial success) increase in psychological importance but become more elusive in reality, antisocial means for obtaining these goals may become more accepted, covertly and implicitly if not overtly and explicitly. Corruption, violence, and other antisocial behavior may be increasingly accepted means for obtaining socially approved goals. The perception of antisocial behavior as pervasive and unavoidably necessary to achieve one's ends may disinhibit further antisocial behavior and rationalize its existence. Thus, normative standards are further weakened and antisocial behavior is perpetuated in a vicious cycle.

In a test of Merton's hypothesis that crime is the result of anomic deviancy, Stack (S. Stack, "Homicide and Property Crime: The Relationship to Anomie," *Aggressive Behavior*, 9(4):339–344 [1983]) found that income inequality significantly predicted homicide, but not property crimes, in 50 of the United States and in 20 other nations. Income inequality represents a state in which individuals may perceive a gap between a cultural goal (i.e., financial success) and cultural methods for obtaining financial success. The results suggest that such a gap may produce frustration leading to aggression.

Anomie, which is significantly and positively related to people's perception of adverse changes in their personal financial status (M. Boor, "Anomie and United States Suicide Rates, 1976," *Journal of Clinical Psychology*, 35(4):703–706

[1979]; M. Boor, "Relationship of Anomie to Perceived Changes in Financial Status, 1973–1980," *Journal of Clinical Psychology*, 38(4):891–892 [1982]), may predispose certain people to antisocial behavior. Edwards (D. W. Edwards, "Sex Role Attitudes, Anomy, and Female Criminal Behavior," *Corrective and Social Psychiatry and Journal of Behavior Technology, Methods, Therapy*, 28(1):14 [1982]) found that anomie is associated with criminal behavior in women.

Mothers who abuse their children have significantly greater anomie than those who do not (C. Shorkey and J. Armendariz, "Personal Worth, Self-Esteem, Anomia, Hostility, and Irrational Thinking of Abusing Mothers: A Multivariate Approach," *Journal of Clinical Psychology*, 41(3):414–421 [1985]). Abuse may facilitate psychopathy in children with certain personal dispositions (e.g., attention deficits). Anomie is significantly associated with alcoholism (D. Albas, C. Albas, and K. W. McCluskey, "Anomie, Social Class, and Drinking Behavior of High School Students," *Journal of Studies on Alcohol*, 39(5):910–913 [1978]), which is a characteristic of many psychopaths. However, anomie is positively associated with suicide, whereas psychopaths seldom commit suicide.

Seeman (M. Seeman, "Alienation Studies," *Annual Review of Sociology*, 1:91–124 [1975]) has proposed a multidimensional social psychological model of alienation. These dimensions may be stated in terms of social learning theory.

1. *Powerlessness*. The individual expects that he or she will have no control over the consequences of his or her behavior. For example, the individual may expect that his or her political participation is useless.
2. *Normlessness*. The individual believes that it is necessary for him or her and for others to violate explicit norms in order to obtain rewards or avoid punishment. For example, an individual may feel that exaggeration of a resume is necessary to obtain a job.
3. *Meaninglessness*. The individual is not able to predict the consequences of his or her behavior because he or she does not fully comprehend social reality.
4. *Social isolation*. The individual fails to interact with others because he or she does not share their values or norms. Thus, other people do not reinforce or model the behavior that the individual has previously learned.
5. *Cultural estrangement*. The individual does not share the norms and values of others because of his or her socialization in a culture or subculture different from these others.
6. *Self-estrangement*. The individual's behavior is dependent on the anticipation of future rewards in association with an absence of present rewards. The individual may be alienated by performing labor that he or she finds unfulfilling.

Such circumstances produce discrepancy between an individual's real and ideal self-concept. These dimensions of alienation may constitute an increasingly prevalent and adaptive generalized psychopathic tendency. Manderscheid, Silbergeld, and Dager (1975) have created a systems model that causally relates social structure, physiological stress, alienation, and perceptual style. In their model, social structural stressors (e.g., minority status, low socioeconomic status) produce both psychological and "physiobiochemical" stress. Psychological stress produces cognitive alienation, as represented by Seeman's alienation dimensions, which serves to reduce psychological stress. Physiobiochemical stress produces affective alienation, represented by Gottschalk's hostility categories, which serves to reduce physiobiochemical stress. Cognitive and affective alienation produce dimensions of perceptual style related to specific types of alienation. For example, powerlessness will produce high perceived submission and low perceived autonomy. Manderscheid et al. propose that the reduction of alienation must involve changes on both an individual and social level.

17. G. Bateson, *Mind and Nature: A Necessary Unity* (New York: Dutton, 1979).
18. Ibid.
19. C. E. Osgood, "A Dinosaur Caper: Psycholinguistics, Past, Present and Future," in D. Aaronson and R. W. Rieber (Eds.), *Developmental Psycholinguistics and Communicative Disorders*, Annals of the New York Academy of Sciences, 263:16–26, 1975).
20. J. Fisher, *The A.P.A. Monitor* (Washington, DC: American Psychological Association, April 1984).
21. R. Merton, "Three Fragments from a Sociologist's Notebooks," *The Annual Review of Sociology*, 13:8–10 (1987).
22. The behavior produced by partial learned helplessness and low cortical arousal may reflect dissociative reactions, such as depersonalization, in which the person develops a sense of himself and others as objects. Depersonalization is often a dissociative reaction that acts as a defense against trauma and anxiety in accident victims and psychiatric patients (R. Noyes and R. Kletti, "Depersonalization in the Face of Life-Threatening Danger: A Description," *Psychiatry*, 39(1):19–27 (1976]). The socialization of the psychopath commonly involves traumatic experiences (W. McCord, *The Psychopath and Milieu Therapy* [New York: Free Press, 1982]) that may condition the psychopath to respond to stress with dissociation. Thus, dissociation may defend the psychopath against the aversive experience of his or her antisocial behavior (e.g., fear and guilt).

Depersonalization is a dissociative reaction to which the psychopath may be especially susceptible. According to Levy and Wachtel (J. S. Levy and P. L. Wachtel, "Depersonalization: An Effort at Clarification," *American Journal of Psychoanalysis*, 38(4):291–300 [1978]), the two basic features of depersonalization are a sense of "splitting off" from one's actions and one's self (i.e., depersonalization) and a sense of unreality about one's self or about objects (i.e., derealization). Depersonalization and derealization were found to be independent factors, each reflecting a transient state that, when measured by self report was positively correlated with anxiety and depression, but that when assessed by diagnostic interview was not correlated with anxiety and depression. See J. L. Fleiss, B. J. Gurland, and B. Goldberg, "Independence of Depersonalization-derealization" *Journal of Consulting and Clinical Psychology*, 43(1):110–111 (1975).

The psychopath may be more susceptible to depersonalization than to derealization. Dorr and Woodhall (D. Dorr, and P. Woodhall, "Ego Dysfunction in Psychopathic Inpatients," in W. H. Reid, D. Dorr, J. I. Walker, and J. W. Bonner, [Eds.], *Unmasking the Psychopath,* [New York: Norton, 1986], pp. 98–131) found that psychopaths were above average in their sense of the reality of the world, but deficient in their sense of the reality of themselves (e.g., body image, self-esteem, individuality). Further, they found that psychopaths were deficient in reality testing (e.g., the accuracy of perceptions of the self and of external events) and in judgment (e.g., the correct anticipation of consequences). Dorr and Woodhall observe that the psychopath's contact with external reality is distorted, selective, and amnesic when it concerns his or her drives and needs, despite his or her hypervigilance to certain stimuli.

Controversy (M. Orne, D. Dinges, E. C. Orne, "On the Differential Diagnosis of Multiple Personality in the Forensic Context," *International Journal of Clinical and Experimental Hypnosis,* 32(2):118–169 [1984]; J. Watkins, "The Bianchi (L.A. Hillside Strangler) Case: Sociopath or Multiple Personality," *International Journal of Clinical and Experimental Hypnosis,* 32(2):67–101 [1984]) has surrounded whether or not K. Bianchi, the "Hillside Strangler," had a multiple personality disorder or an APD plus sexual sadism. While the interpretations of the facts in the Bianchi case are not conclusive, the case raises the possibility that the psychopath may exercise dissociative ability in the performance of antisocial behavior. Bianchi's fraudulent malingering would itself represent an exercise of an ability to dissociate himself from his crimes, if not a true multiple personality.

Empirical studies have recently begun to indirectly approach the issue of the dissociative capacity of the psychopath. Psychopaths do relatively poorly on tasks requiring divided attention; that is, they do not "overfocus" on one task to the exclusion of a second simultaneous task. See D. S. Kosson and J. P. Newman, "Psychopathy and the Allocation of Attentional Capacity in a Divided-Attention Situation," *Journal of Abnormal Psychology,* 95(3):257–263 (1986). Kosson and Newman state that their evidence contradicts their hypothesis that psychopaths will overfocus on immediate goals to the exclusion of long-term consequences. However, the fact that psychopaths are poor in divided attention tasks may be interpreted as a due to a disposition to absorption that impairs their ability to divide their attention. Also, the reaction time tasks used by Kosson and Newman may have been inappropriate for psychopathic subjects because such individuals have innately low levels of cortical arousal, which may confound the effects of the attentional manipulation. In fact, Kosson and Newman found that psychopaths had particularly slow reaction times, also possibly due to their low levels of autonomic arousal. Smith (R. J. Smith, *The Psychopath in Society* [New York: Academic Press, 1978]) has noted that the use of stimulus materials that lower the already deficient arousal of the psychopath produces confounded and artifactual results, and are a common fallacy in experimental studies of psychopaths. According to the model formulated by Spiegel (H. Spiegel, "The Hypnotic Induction Profile (HIP): A Review of its Development," *Annals of the New York Academy of Sciences,* 296:129–142 [1977]; H. Spiegel and D. Spiegel, *Trance and Treatment: The Clinical Uses of Hypnosis,* [New

York: Basic Books, 1978]), absorption is a biologically based disposition that promotes hypnotizability. Absorption produces intense concentration and is mediated by socialization and conditioning to produce a personality style characterized by an orientation centered in immediate temporal and spatial perception. The biological potential for absorption can be measured by such indices as Eye Roll using the Hypnotic Induction Profile (HIP). The absorption of consciousness into a specific experience produces dissociation in which consciousness is divided into separate complexes. Absorption and dissociation are the preconditions for the heightened suggestibility that produces compliance because inhibitions upon impulses are dissociated from consciousness while suggestions are given focused attention. According to Spiegel, the pathological person has a greater capacity for absorption than he or she can utilize, as indicated by broken concentration on the HIP.

In our opinion, psychopaths' biological capacity for absorption may be heavily utilized by them because they are conditioned by their socialization to become absorbed in the stimulation produced by reward and its expectation while becoming dissociated from the aversive experience produced by punishment and its expectation. Thus, psychopaths may become so absorbed in the rewarding stimulation produced by antisocial behavior that they dissociate from the aversive consequences of their antisocial behavior. Psychopaths' absorption and dissociation prevent them from fully attending to the aversive consequences of antisocial behavior, both for themselves and for others. Full attention to such aversive consequences would otherwise inhibit the performance of antisocial behavior by provoking guilt and fear. Further, dissociation may disinhibit psychopaths' performance of the antisocial behavior that is motivated by their innate disposition to seek stimulation to compensate their deficient cortical arousal.

Furthermore, we think that Spiegel's model may provide a more detailed explanation of psychopaths' lack of guilt and empathy in terms of dissociation, specifically their selective amnesia and defensive rationalization. Psychopaths dissociate from the negative affective experiences (e.g., guilt) entailed in their actions through selective amnesia. This affective amnesia facilitates psychopaths' cognitive rationalization of their behavior in response to external pressure (e.g., interrogation). Such rationalizations may further defend the psychopath from experiencing the guilt that might otherwise be evoked to disinhibit further antisocial behavior. The apparent absence of affect and anxiety in the primary psychopath may be the result of dissociation, which functions to defend him or her from anxiety.

According to Doren (D. M. Doren, *Understanding and Treating the Psychopath*, [New York: Wiley, 1987]), the psychopath is disposed to risk-taking by his or her partial learned helplessness and innately low cortical arousal. Situations that provide unpredictable reinforcement and punishment may be particularly effective in disinhibiting the behavior of the psychopath.

23. L. Festinger, H. W. Reicken, and S. Schacter, *When Prophecy Fails* (Minneapolis: University of Minnesota Press, 1956).

24. The fact that incarcerated psychopaths can have psychotic breakdowns has

been repeatedly observed over many years especially where and when gross solitary confinement procedures were prevalent in prisons. This unusual induced psychotic breakdown should be distinguished from the Ganser state first described in the nineteenth century as a mental disease in which the inmate of a prison desires to be perceived innocent so he may be pardoned and fakes his behavior for that purpose. During the latter part of the nineteenth century and the early part of the twentieth century, these conditions were referred to as purpose psychoses. Today, we would refer to them as the malingering of psychotic states of mental illness. Bleuer in his famous textbook, *Psychiatry*, refers to these conditions as situational psychosis. It is not uncommon to see incarcerated psychopaths engage in malingering illnesses and/or beneficial effects from treatment for the purposes of secondary gain.

25. H. S. Sullivan, *Interpersonal Theory of Psychiatry* (New York: Norton, 1953) p. 360.
26. For an interesting study of this behavior during World War II, see H. S. Ripley and S. Wolf, "Psychoses Occurring among Psychopathic Personalities in Association with Inelastic Situations Overseas," *American Journal of Psychiatry*, 105:52–59 (1948).
27. We have no intention to suggest in this remark that psychopathy is caused by abuse during childhood. Although from a clinical point of view experience has illustrated ample evidence that there is a correlation between psychopathy and various degrees of abuse during childhood, no direct cause can be assumed from a correlation.
28. Eysenck views psychopathy as a genetically determined disposition both to low cortical arousal (i.e., extraversion) and to high sympathetic nervous system arousal (i.e., neuroticism) that prevents the learning of appropriate responses (e.g., fear in response to punishment). Eysenck's theory, like Gough 's theory, has been criticized because research based on it has been limited to criminal populations. Thus, the theory may refer more to criminality than to psychopathy. Also, the reliability and validity of the scales composing the Eysenck Personality Inventory used to measure extraversion, neuroticism, and psychoticism have been seriously questioned.

    Studies indicating that the brain waves of psychopaths, as measured by electroencephalogram (EEG), are slower than those of normal individuals strongly support the contention that the disposition to low cortical arousal (i.e., extraversion) is characteristic of the psychopath. However, evidence that psychopaths are more emotionally reactive (i.e., neurotic) is contradictory, and overwhelmingly suggests that psychopaths, to the contrary, are less emotionally reactive than normal individuals. Experimental evidence indicates that psychopaths are deficient in the classical conditioning of emotional reactions compared to normal subjects. Psychopaths are also deficient in instrumentally conditioned avoidance of punishment. Under conditions of uncertain punishment, psychopaths will persist at simple tasks more than normals, especially if the possibility of positive reinforcement exists. Some evidence suggests that psychopaths are more adept at observational learning and imitation that involve perceived gain and social reinforcement. Overall, Eysenck's contention avoidance compared to normals is well supported. Contrary to Eysenck's theory, psychopaths have been found to learn as well or better than normals in certain conditions.

Hare (R. D. Hare, *Psychopathy: Theory and Research*, [New York: Wiley, 1970]) has postulated that the psychopath suffers from lesions in the limbic system that cause a loss of inhibition and a preservation of their dominant responses, which are characteristically antisocial. Animal studies have indicated that lesions in the limbic system of animals can produce the preservation of dominant (i.e., well-learned) responses, even in inappropriate situations. However, these animals eventually learn new responses.

Most criminal psychopaths have been estimated to have abnormally slow brain wave patterns, but these patterns are not indicative of organic disorder. Also, some researchers have questioned the existence and meaning of abnormal brain wave activity. Psychopaths have a greater than normal incidence of organic brain syndromes, but not necessarily in limbic system disorders. Hare's theory is intended to account only for the response preservation of psychopaths.

The abnormally high slow-wave activity of the psychopath, which indicates low cortical arousal, suggests that psychopaths suffer from a "maturational lag" that produces egocentricity, impulsivity, and an inability to delay gratification. Psychopaths eventually "burn out" as they reach middle age; that is, they decrease or terminate their antisocial behavior. Kegan (Kegan, "The Child behind the Mask: Sociopathy as Developmental Delay," in W. Reid et al. [Eds.], *Unmasking the Psychopath* [New York: Norton, 1986], p. 45–77) has proposed that the psychopath does not generally develop beyond preconventional moral reasoning, which is oriented exclusively toward external rewards and punishments. However, not all individuals (approximately 15 percent of the population) who manifest a similar brain wave pattern are socially deviant. Also, the psychopath possesses many characteristics that are not typical of the average child, although the similarity in moral reasoning of children and psychopaths make maturational retardation a compelling analogy.

29. F. Redl and D. Wineman, *Children Who Hate* (New York: Free Press, 1951).
30. In a recent book by Sommers, the story of the life of J. Edgar Hoover provides a chilling example of a psychopath who was in such a high position of power that he managed to escape exposure during his lifetime. For over 40 years he managed to corrupt one of the most important institutions within the government, the Federal Bureau of Investigation, cheat the taxpayers, and protect criminals in high places including many mafia leaders.

CHAPTER 3

1. It may be of some value to remember Nietzsche's observations on war and peace:

   And perhaps the great day will come when a people, distinguished by wars and victories and by the highest development of a military order and intelligence, and accustomed to make the heaviest sacrifices for these things, will exclaim of its own free will, "We break the sword, and will smash its entire military establishment down to its lowest foundations. Rendering oneself unarmed when one has been the best armed, out of a height of feeling that this is the means to a real peace, which must always rest on a peace of mind: whereas the so-called armed peace, as it now exists in all countries, is the absence of peace of mind. One trusts neither oneself nor one's neighbor and, half from hatred, half from fear, does not lay down arms. Rather perish than hate and fear, and twice rather perish than make oneself hated and feared—this must someday become the highest maxim for every single commonwealth, too. (*The Wanderer and His Shadow*, p. 204)

2. A. Adler, *The Neurotic Constitution* (New York: Moffat & Yard, 1917).
3. E. Fromm, *The Sane Society* (New York: Bantam Books, 1956).
4. C. G. Jung, *Two Essays in Analytic Psychology* (Princeton: Bollington Press, 1972).
5. W. Trotter, *The Herd Instinct in Times of Peace and War* (New York: McMillan, 1916).
6. K. Goldstein, *The Organism* (New York: American Book, 1939).
7. G. Bateson, *Steps To an Ecology of Mind* (Northvale, NJ: Jason Aronson, 1987).
8. S. Keen, *Faces of the Enemy* (New York: Harper and Row, 1986).
9. T. Sheehan, *The First Coming* (New York: Random House, 1986).
10. F. Redl et al., "Dehumanization," in N. Sanford and C. Comstock (Eds.), *Sanctions for Evil* (San Francisco: Jossey Bass, 1971).
11. R. J. Lifton, *Home from the War* (New York: Simon & Schuster, 1973).
12. R. J. Lifton, "Existential Evil," in N. Sanford and C. Comstock (Eds.) *Sanctions for Evil* (San Francisco: Jossey Bass, 1971).
13. E. Goffman, *Frame Analysis* (New York: Harper, 1974).
14. M. Foucault, *Discipline and Punishment: The Birth of the Prison* (New York: Vintage, 1979).
15. E. Erikson, *Gandhi's Truth* (New York: Norton, 1969), p. 431.
16. V. I. Lenin, *Lenin on the Material and Colonial Questions* (Peking: Foreign Language Press, 1970).

CHAPTER 4

1. The issue of defining deviancy in different ways has become an interesting concern as of late. Crabhammer's notion of defining deviancy "up," in contrast to Senator Patrick Moynihan's notion of defining deviancy "down," addresses the issue of political correctness that places emphasis upon such issues as date rape, academic policing of the use of epithets, false memory syndrome, and child abuse. Crabhammer's notion is that we are creating deviancy where deviancy does not and should not exist. Moynihan's notion is that we are redefining deviancy by playing it down and accepting things that not only should not exist but that also are detrimental to society's welfare (as mentioned in Chapter 2, we have a tendency to downplay the negativism associated with crime, in that it is

no longer seen as a crime to be a criminal). Such things would include the general disintegration of the family (particularly the widespread acceptance of children being born out of wedlock), which holds relevance to our discussion of the causative factors associated with the psychopathy of everyday life.

Really, the business of defining deviancy "up" or "down" is dependent upon where the person who is doing the defining is standing; in either instance, what is occurring here is deviancy being defined "away." These observations, in my opinion, are best understood as symptoms of society's rapid social transformation, which is part and parcel of the processes of social distress and the psychopathy of everyday life, which grows out of the social distress syndrome.

Moynihan offers three categories of redefinition: (1) altruistic (i.e., redistribution of mental health services); (2) opportunistic (i.e., acceptance of alternative family structures); and (3) normalizing (i.e., acceptance of unprecedented levels of violent crime).

These three categories are descibed as an "interactive" process, reciprocally affecting one another. Moynihan provides a lot of documented evidence to support his contention. See D. P. Moynihan, "Defining deviancy Down," *American Educator*, Winter 1993–94, 12–18; C. Crabhammer, "White-Collar Crime," *New Republic*, November 22, 1993.

2. A classic category of criminal activity was referred to as white-collar crime. Criminologists who wrote about it rarely managed to plumb the depths of character of the white-collar criminal, probably because they were mostly sociologists. If one looks back 50 years or so at white-collar crime and criminals, they are remarkably similar to today's offenses and offenders. See H. J. Vetter and L. Territo, *Crime and Practice in America* (St. Paul: West Publishing, 1984), pp. 12–13.

3. Noam Chomsky's work relating to the media, as well as other political works, provides us with ample evidence regarding this matter. Especially pertinent to this is the recently released film about Chomsky's intellectual career, which is appropriately titled *The Manufacturing of Consent*.

4. The Keating S&L scandal is the most alarming case of the hundreds of S&L collapses that have recently taken place, given the circumstances leading up to the bank's bailout in 1989. Keating purchased the Lincoln Savings and Loan Association for $51 million in 1984. He went beyond the traditional procedures for S&L institutions, taking advantage of the relatively liberal regulations for such banks in the state of California. When depositors came in to buy federally insured certificates of deposit, tellers at Lincoln S&L directed them to sales representatives who sold them junk bonds issued by American Continental, a corporation formed by Keating. The Federal Home Loan Bank in San Francisco began an investigation of Lincoln's growth and investment activities during 1986 and urged Washington to examine the case, since they found that Lincoln was operating under questionable loan and accounting practices.

In September 1990, Keating was charged by a state grand jury for duping investors into buying junk bonds. During the trial, which lasted nearly a month, depositors, many of them elderly, said that they were not fully informed of the riskiness of the bonds and that they did not fully understand that the bonds were not federally insured. On December 4, 1991, Keating was finally found guilty of securities fraud. His defense attorney, Stephen C. Neal, contended that the prosecution had "utterly failed" to prove that Keating had engaged in criminal activity, since all the risks pertaining to the bonds sold to the depositors were fully explained in the prospectus given to the buyers.

For a further discussion of the S&L scandal, see S. Pizzo and P. Muolo, "Take the Money and Run: A Rogues' Gallery of Some Lucky S.& L. Thieves," *New York Times Magazine*, May 9, 1993).

5. Ibid.
6. A good example of this is the most recent terrorist attack in early 1993 when terrorists planted a bomb in the World Trade Center and caused panic and death in New York City's financial district.
7. See Moynihan's discussion on the effect of the interest group rewards derived from the acceptance of alternative family structures. D. P. Moynihan, "Defining Deviancy Down," *American Educator*, Winter 1993–94, 12–18.
8. Another example of this was seen in spring of 1993 in the difficulty the United Nations experienced in their attempts to bring food into the war torn areas of Somalia. More often than not, the food never reached the people for whom it was intended.
9. In his discussion pertaining to Jim and Tammy Bakker, Saxe further provides the reader with additional insight into the ubiquitous nature of the phenomenon known as the psychopathy of everyday life. Saxe says, "Recent history has not spared even religious leaders from involvement in scandal and deceit. From the Reverend Jim Bakker, convicted of fraud, to Reverend Jimmy Swaggart, found to have engaged prostitutes while proselytizing against the evils of sex, examples of destructive deceptiveness abound." L. Saxe, "Lying: Thoughts of an Applied Social Psychologist," *American Psychologist*, 46(4):409–415.

CHAPTER 5

1. This lyric, like the one in *Thunderball*, reveals an important theme in the James Bond movie saga. First, dreams are for sale and you've got to pay for them. Second, you make your wishes come true by acting them out. And third, you've got to be a "doppelganger," i.e., dissociate or divide your consciousness, in order to act out your dreams.
2. It is of interest to add here the fact that adults acquire—or understand—the more abstract aspects of a natural language, such as syntax, semantics, and pragmatics, while children are better with the acquisition of lexical items and phonological rules. For example, an adult would more easily recognize the meaning in context of a regularly conjugated verb, whereas a child would be more prone to remembering and pronouncing correctly an irregular verb.
3. The Jungian notion of archetypes is very similar to the idea we are introducing of the universal symbol. Our interpretation of dreams, however, does not necessarily coincide with that of Jung.
4. The Freudian interpretation of dreams, one of the best-known theories, ex-

plains the function of dreams as a way for individuals to express and fulfill certain unconscious wishes that come from repressed thoughts believed by the individual to be unacceptable. This more restrictive interpretation, however, does not constitute the frame of reference we wish to use in our interpretation of dreams.

5. Lakoff discusses how the unconscious metaphor system helps to structure thought processes as well as dream processes. For further information see G. Lakoff, "How Metaphors Structure Dreams," *Dreaming*, 3(2):77–98.

6. Ernst Cassirer, *The Philosophy of Symbolic Forms*, (New York: Yale University Press, 1959).

7. L. Frank, *Individual Development* (New York: Random House, 1955).

8. We may conceive of the dream process, or "work," as Freud called it, as the type of event that is not so, at least in the form that it is given to us. What the dream language means is to be found or interpreted in the process that was developed first in the dream itself (i.e., the story) and in the unfolding dialectic process, which includes the interpersonal as well as the broader social context involved in the interpretation.

9. My interpretation of the collective unconscious does not adhere to specific assumptions made by Jung.

10. "In der ganzen Geschiechte des Menschen ist kein Kapitel unterrichtender fur Herz und Geist als die Annalen seiner Verirrungen." *Der Verbrecher aus Verlorener Ehre.*

11. E. Said, *Culture and Imperialism* (New York: Random House, 1983).

12. T. S. Elliott, from "The Wind Sprang up at Four O'Clock."

13. It would prove almost impossible to create here a complete catalogue of all social dreams portraying the theme of social distress and institutionalized psychopathy. The following, however, deserve honorable mention as social dreams quite pertinent to but not included in our discussion. The very popular films about the Mafia, from *Godfather* to the most recent *Goodfellas*, depict the problem of institutionalized distress quite clearly. The Jack Lemmon film *Save the Tiger*, about an industrial garment merchant and manufacturer in New York City, also conveys our theme of interest, as the merchant is trapped by social distress into becoming an arsonist to save his business. The film *Bonfire of the Vanities*, based on the very popular book of the same title, also unveiled the problems related to social distress, especially at the end when a black judge accuses the entire chamber of unethical deeds and irresponsibility. Finally, another social dream we must mention is the film *Pacific Heights*. It is the story of a young unmarried couple that invests in an apartment only to be victimized by the tenant, a psychopath who drives them to violence. The law goes on the side of the psychopath, forcing the victimized couple to become psychopaths in order to survive. This problem, driving normal people to vigilante tactics, was the main subject matter for the Charles Bronson films. The psychopath uses the law in his favor, and the trusting victims, who try to do the common decent thing, are driven to take the other more violent and unlawful action, only to be convicted in the end.

14. *Metropolis* was a UFA film made in Germany during the 1920s. It depicts a

futuristic ultracomputerized society where the easy manipulation of the masses takes place by means of information media.

15. See Chapter 6 for a further discussion.

16. In Stone's rather surrealistic and futuristic film, the question as to what the mind understands as real in the world is played with as a theme that interacts with high technology and manipulation of the minds of human beings and the world that they live in.

17. Written in the 1950s, a book by Philip Wiley, *The Disappearance*, presents a nightmarish social dream about the self-defeating battle of the sexes. On a certain unhappy day, all women disappear and exist in a parallel world to that of the men. In both worlds, the separate sexes must deal with the outcome and devise ways to survive.

18. The media has announced that in order to keep up with the times and be politically correct, Superman will be transformed into a many splendored thing—the multicultural Superman. The question still remains, where will it all end? Clearly, a multicultural Superman reflects the spirit of the times, where not only does the hyphenated American claim victim status but also needs its antithesis status—Superman status—to make up for it.

19. "Katzenjammer" in German means hangover.

CHAPTER 6

1. Discussions on the trials of the World Trade Center bombers, their organization and objectives, may be found in Robert J. Kelly, "The Politics of Atrocity and the Cult of Counterterrorism," Parts I and II, *Magazin fur die Polizei*, 23(198, 199) (Oct./Nov. 1992) and R. J. Kelly, "Guilty: The Verdict against Terror in the World Trade Center Bombing," *Magazin fur die Polizei*, 25 (July/August 1994).

2. J. D. Simon, *The Terrorist Trap: America's Experience with Terrorism* (Bloomington: Indiana University Press, 1994).

3. I. Cohn and G. S. Gordon-Gill, in J. Goldberg, "A War Without Purpose," *New York Times Magazine*, January 22, 1995, pp. 36–40. *Child Soldiers* (Geneva: Institut Henry-Dunant). T. Rosenberg, *Children of Cain: Violence and the Violent in Latin America* (New York: Morrow, 1991).

4. B. M. Jenkins, *Future Trends in International Terrorism* (Santa Monica, CA: The Rand Corporation, 1985), p. 7176. R. J. Kelly and W. Cook, "Experience in International Travel and Aversion to Terrorism," *Journal of Police and Criminal Psychology*, 10(2) (April 1994).

5. K. L. Adelman and N. R. Augustine, *The Defense Revolution: Intelligent Downsizing of America's Military* (San Francisco: Institute for Contemporary Studies, 1990).

6. Space limitations preclude a discussion of chemical and biological weapons that are quite lethal, readily available, and easier to handle than nuclear weapons. Among states that have resorted to chemical agents, Iraq has been the most blatant during its war against Iran in the 1980s and against Kurdish rebels in Northern Iraq.

7. A. Speer, *Inside the Third Reich* (New York: Knopf, 1982).
8. On the issue of changing social identities where sex, gender, ethnicity and race replace class notions, see Stanley Aronowitz, *Roll Over Beethoven: The Return of Cultural Strife* (Hanover, New Hampshire: Wesleyan University Press, 1993), and William W. Zellner, *Countercultures: A Sociological Analysis* (New York: St. Martin's Press, 1995), for discussion on marginal and irredentist nativist movements that are transnational in scope and aspiration.
9. R. J. Kelly, "Political Crimes and the Emergence of Revolutionary Nationalist Ideologies," in R. S. Denisoff and C. McCaghy, (Eds.) *Deviance, Conflict and Criminality*, Chicago: Rand McNally, (1973). R. J. Kelly, "From Pistols to Ploughshares: The IRA's Farewell to Arms," *International Journal of Comparative and Applied Criminal Justice* 20(1):106 (1995).
10. Mark Hagopian, *The Phenomenon of Revolution* (New York: Dodd, Mead, 1974); Albert Parry, *Terrorism from Robespierre to Arafat* (New York: Vanguard Press, 1976); Richard Pipes, *The Russian Revolution* (New York: Alfred A. Knopf, 1990), Ch. 8. These writers suggest that terrorism practiced by states was not an isolated, fortuitous—even if recurrent—expression of a government's exasperation but a system: a plan for mass intimidation, compulsion, and murder. In the hands of government agencies operating clandestinely, terror is a deliberately calculated response to challenges, real or imagined (and the latter too frequently illustrates the paranoia rampant in a regime), where punitive activities including assassination, exile, incarceration, informal reprisals, the suppression of free speech and criticism, the ubiquity of police agents and informers, and the violation of human rights create an apparatus of repression that has durability and never ceases to function, going on intermittently at varying levels of intensity throughout the life of a regime.

In contrast to the Jacobin Terror of 1793–94, according to Pipes, the Bolshevik Terror emanated not from below but from the Politburo permanently chaired by Lenin himself. Pipes's anti-Leninist zeal blinds him to authoritative accounts of the French Reign of Terror where not individuals but bureaucracy and laws initiated the violence. Furet, for instance, thinks that the bloodletting was unleashed by the Law of 22 Prairial—the Law of Suspects—which later consumed most of The Committee of Public Safety and the Republicans who supported its extremist repressions. See Francois Furet, *Interpreting the French Revolution*, trans. E. Forster (New York: Cambridge University Press, 1989); Georges Lefebvre, *The Thermidorians*, trans. Robert Baldick (New York: Vintage Books). Indeed, on examination of state-sponsored terror across the historical sweep of great transformative revolutionary movements in the Russian, French and Chinese cases—especially the Cultural Revolution and "Great Leap Forward" inaugurated by Mao, it becomes evident that (1) they are principally focused on the key enemy—the people themselves—and (2) the apparatus for the repression is a mix of party officials, military, and police cadres. In this connection, see Richard M. Pfeffer, "Mao Tse-Tung and the Cultural Revolution" in Norman Miller and Roderick Aya (Eds.), *National Liberation: Revolution in the Third World* (New York: Free Press, 1971). Pfeffer, in spite of himself, describes how Mao set in motion widespread terror against the Chinese masses through his mobilization of party cadres and youth. Though they were directed to carry out purges of party elites, bureaucrats, and party opponents, not surprisingly it was the peasants who felt the brunt of the repression.

11. J. Inciardi, "Narcoterrorism: A Perspective and Commentary," in Robert J. Kelly and Donal E. J. MacNamara (Eds.), *Perspectives on Deviance* (Cincinnati, OH: Anderson Publishing, 1991).

12. M. S. Steinitz, "Insurgents, Terrorists and the Drug Trade," *The Washington Quarterly*, Fall 1985.

13. R. W. Lee, III, "Colombia's Cocaine Syndicates," in Alfred W. McCoy and Alan Block (Eds.), *War on Drugs* (Boulder, CO: Westview Press, 1992).

14. R. J. Kelly, "Breaking the Seals of Silence: Anti-Mafia Uprising in Sicily," *USA Today Magazine*, July 1994.

15. P. Williams, "Transnational Criminal Organizations and International Security," *Survival*, 36(1) (Spring 1994).

16. J. O. Finckenauer, "Russian Organized Crime in America," in Robert J. Kelly, Ko-lin Chin, and Rufus Schatzberg (Eds.), *Handbook of Organized Crime in the United States* (Westport, CT: Greenwood Press, 1994).

17. D. E. Kaplan and A. Dubro, *Yakuza* (Reading, MA: Addison-Wesley, 1986); C. Sterling, *Thieves' World: The Threat of the New Global Network of Organized Crime* (New York: Simon and Schuster, 1994).

18. C Sterling, *Thieves' World*, pp. 14–15.

19. In specifically addressing the international nature of organized crime, the United Nations Economic and Social Council observed that:

International experience shows that organized crime has long ago crossed national borders and is today transnational.... It should be noted that aspects of the evolutionary process undergone by society may make powerful criminal organizations even more impenetrable and facilitate the expansion of their illegal activities. (United Nations, Report of the Commission on Crime Prevention and Criminal Justice on Its First Session, *Substantive Session of the Economic and Social Council*, Vienna, Austria, 1992, p. 32)

20. When Alexander Solzhenitsyn returned to Russia two years ago he planned to travel by train from Vladivostok in the East to Moscow in order to get a feel of the mood of the country. Somewhere east of the Urals in the Donets region, racketeers stopped the train demanding a "fee." It was only through the intervention of high officials and the mobilization of regional police that he was able to proceed unmolested by extortionists.

21. J. Holder-Rhodes and P. A. Lupsha, "Gray Area Phenomena: New Threats and Policy Dilemmas," *CJ. International*, 9(1) (January-February 1993); National Strategy Information Center, *The Gray Area Phenomenon: Report of a Research Seminar* (July) (1992). (Washington, DC).

22. R. J. Kelly and K. Chin, "Illegal Chinese Immigrants and Smuggling Rings," *National Science Foundation, Report* (1995).

23. In this connection, Aristotle has some useful insight. Commenting on types of government and the character of leaders, he says:

When speaking of royalty we also spoke of two forms of tyranny, which are both according to law, and therefore easily pass into royalty. Among Barbarians there are elected monarchs who exercise a despotic power; despotic rulers were also elected in ancient Hellas, called Aesymnetes or dictators. There monarchies, when compared with one another, exhibit certain differences. And they are, as I said before, royal, in so far as the monarch rules according to law over willing subjects; but they are tyrannical in so far as he is despotic and rules according to his own fancy. There is also a third kind of tyranny, which is the most typical form, and is the counterpart of the perfect monarchy. This tyranny is just that arbitrary power of an individual which is responsible to no one, and governs all alike, whether equals or better, with a view to its own advantage, not to that of its subjects, and therefore against their will. No freeman, if he can escape from it, will endure such a government. The kinds of tyranny are such and so many, and for the reasons for which I have given. (Aristotle, *The Politics* (New York: Oxford University Press, 1941) II, 219.

24. J. B. Elshtain, *Democracy on Trial* (New York: Basic Books, 1995).
25. M. Van Crevald, *The Transformation of War* (New York: Free Press, 1991).
26. Ibid., 193.
27. In looking for parallels with the right-wing militia movements spreading in rural white America, mainly in the states west of the Mississippi, some similarities with urban groups are apparent. First, the wariness of federal law enforcement agencies (FBI, ATF) and the criticism of their high-handedness in dealing with ordinary citizens are matched by community suspicions and misgivings about local police forces in the racial ghettos of most large American cities. Second, in addition to the fear promoted by law enforcement the motives behind the formation of the movement may be no different in essence than those that led to urban crime families and street gangs; in short, the Arizona Patriots and Michigan Militia are matched, as it were, by the Crips and Bloods of Los Angeles.

CHAPTER 7

1. As early as 1863 a booklet was anonymously published for popular consumption to warn the general public about the current humbuggery that had already become institutionalized within the culture. Most of it appears very much like the psychopathy of everyday life we encounter today. For example, the advertising, swindling, quacks, the subscription cons through the mail, how to make a quick fortune con, the gift business swindle, the lottery games, and the phoney drug con. See *Humbug: A Look at Some Popular Impositions* (New York: S.F. French, 1863). There is an interesting parallel to this nineteenth century example in the telemarketing scams in the early part of the 1990s.

Over a hundred years later, in 1938, Joseph Jastrow, one of the original popularizers of psychology and already famous for his activity in exposing swindlers and the like, had this to say about the American national character:

Plainly, the betrayal of intelligence extends far beyond adviseering and sales-manship. It enters into the temper and texture of the American way of thinking, our ideology. Much of our enterprise in commodities and ideas, in ponderables and imponderables, thrives in an atmosphere of betrayal. Under such hospitality, the industrial habit of mind is carried over deliberately, as well as by a subconscious momentum, into fields where its pressure creates havoc. The bull, suited to the pasture, wrecks the china shop. The great American fallacy consists in, and insists upon, running as a business what cannot be so managed without sacrificing intrinsic values, in making a business of pursuits dependent upon quite other loyalties, commonly called cultural. The box-office, the cash-register, the promoter are the money-changers in the modern temples. (J. Jastrow, *The Betrayal of Intelligence* [New York: Greenberg, 1938], p. 21).

2. Carl Zimmerman (C. Zimmerman, *The Family of Tomorrow: The Cultural Crisis and the Way Out* [New York: Harper Brothers, 1949]), in discussing the historical roots of the family and the invisible cultural worlds represented in Aristophanes classic *The Clouds*, presents this warning: "The confusion of the invisible cultural world lays an increasing strain upon the individual and causes the development of the psychopathic personality. The rise of the psychopathic personality is another symptom of the disintegration of the family," (p. 68).

3. Baudrillard's position regarding virtual reality and the media in principle is compatible with my point of view, although I do not necessarily agree with the details of his theory. See Jean Baudrillard "Virtual Illusion or the Automatic Writing of the World," *Theory, Culture, and Society*, 12(4):48 (1995).

4. R. J. Lifton, "Protean Man," *Archives of General Psychiatry*, 24:298–304 (1971).

5. C. Geertz, *Local Knowledge: Further Essays on Interpretive Anthropology* (New York: Basic Books, 1983).

6. Mary Douglas [*How Institutions Think* (London: Routledge & Kegan Paul, 1987)] also has some pertinent things to say regarding this principle:

   Institutions systematically direct individual memory and channel our perceptions compatible with the relations they authorize. They fix processes that are essentially dynamic, they hide their influence and they arouse our emotions to a standardized pitch on standardized issues … no wonder they easily recruit us into joining their narcissistic self-contemplation. Any problems we try to think about are automatically transformed into their own organizational problems … if the institution is one that depends on participation, it will reply to our frantic question "more participation!" If it is one that depends on authority it will only reply "more authority!" Institutions have the pathetic megalomania of the computer whose whole vision of the world is its own program. For us the hope of intellectual independence is to resist, the necessary first step in resistance is to understand how the institutional grip affects the mind of the individual.

7. I am in complete agreement with Saxe when he states, "A kind of hysteria about dishonesty seems to have permeated our culture. Perhaps stimulated by pervasive mendacity, we are quick to call others liars and frauds." Furthermore, Saxe believes that

   the need to encourage honesty is clearly pressing. Ways to reinforce honesty need to be found, perhaps even for individuals who have done despicable deeds. Society cannot function well with the massive dishonesty now evident, and increasing the penalties for dishonest behavior may only serve to create additional deception. The effects of rampant dishonesty, from a lack of confidence in governmental leaders to mistrust among colleagues and friends, can only have a corrosive impact on our public lives. (L. Saxe, "Lying: Thoughts of an Applied Social Psychologist," *American Psychologist* 46(4):409–415)

INDEX

207